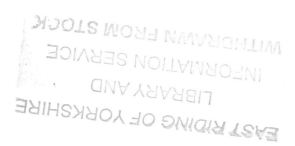

For the Love of Alice

The inspiring story of the
Maddocks family's fight to save their
precious daughter

MALCOLM STACEY
with Dean & Carol Maddocks

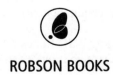

ROBSON BOOKS

First published in Great Britain in 2003 by Robson Books, The Chrysalis Building, Bramley Road, London W10 6SP

A member of **Chrysalis** Books plc

British Library Cataloguing in Publication Data
A catalogue record for this title is available from the British Library.

ISBN 1 86105 605 2

Photo Section Credits
p1 © Sue Ellis; p2 (top left) family album, (top right) family album, (bottom) © Tempest Photography; p3 family album; p4 (top) family album, (bottom) © *Dewsbury Reporter*; p7 (top left) © *Yorkshire Post*, (top right) family album, (bottom) © *Yorkshire Evening Post*; pp 8 and 9 (top left) © West Yorkshire Police, (top centre) family album, (bottom left) © *Yorkshire Evening Post*; (top right) family album, (bottom right) © Downing Street; p10 © *Yorkshire Evening Post*; p12 © PA Photos; p13 © *Yorkshire Post Newspapers*; p14 family album; p15 (top) family album, (bottom) family album; p16 (top left) The 'Press' (Dewsbury), (top right) family album, (centre) family album, (bottom) © Downing Street

Typeset in 11.5pt/14pt Times by FiSH Boooks, London
Printed in Great Britain by Creative Print & Design (Wales) Ebbw Vale

Contents

PART TWO

THIS BOOK IS DEDICATED TO
CHLOE

our beautiful sweet-natured daughter
and Alice's much-loved big sister.

Acknowledgements

Since the day in May 2000 when Alice fell ill our lives have been turned upside down. There have been many times when we have wished we could have our normal life back again. However, we have pulled together and worked as a family to help our younger daughter, Alice, fight for her life. As parents, we have only done what is natural and that is why we go to any length in our desperate fight.

But we could not have got through these times without the large number of kind-hearted people who have given us encouragement, support and prayers over the last three years. We are only able to name a few but we hope that you all know that your kind words, gestures and practical support have undoubtedly helped us get through those dark days.

Firstly we want to thank Malcolm Stacey, without whom none of this would have been possible.

Our wonderful devoted families who look after us with such love and kindness: Mum and Dad Maddocks for the sunshine you bring into Chloe and Alice's lives; Dean's brother, 'The Iron Man' Tony Maddocks and sister-in-law Susan; Pa Lister for your love and encouragement; Carol's late mother, Pat Lister – you taught me how to walk and how to talk, but most of all you taught me how to be strong – you are only ever a prayer away; Carol's very protective brothers – Peter, Paul and David (Baby Face) Lister, and her loving sister and friend, Sue Dymond; Richard Dymond for your wonderful sense of humour; dear Auntie Mary for your gentleness.

Margaret Facer for the constant flow of flowers; Sarah Walsh, our dear and treasured friend, for enriching our lives, 'Our Guardian Angel'; Nigel and Linda for helping us try to understand our computer: ha! ha!; David and Caroline Mullins for your good taste in wine; Arthur King for your introduction to the Rotary Club; Craig Batley for making Alice laugh; Bev Drury who never gives up hope; Tracey Booth-Gibbons, our trusted friend; Lynn and Helen for the laughter and the tears; Alan Pearson, Carol's understanding boss!; Joanne Dickinson for opening your home to Chloe; Inspector Simon Atkin, PS Pat Noon, PC John Cole, PC Simon (marathon man) Woodhead and many others at West Yorkshire Police; the late Craig Scargill and his family; Darren and Claire McKenna for keeping us positive; Mick and Angela (the artist) Hutton; Mike Morris for always making Alice feel at ease; Julie Lockwood; Margaret Emsley; Cathy Stone; Jane Hickson; Christine 'lunch would be lovely' Talbot; Neil Hudson; Sheron Boyle; Liz Rhodes; Neil Hodgkinson; Margaret Watson for your friendship and cake; Christa Ackroyd, Harry Gration; Bryany Detmar of the Aplastic Anaemia Trust – you really do know what we are going through; Professor Ted Gordon Smith for your total dedication to finding a cure for aplastic anaemia; the Governor Stacey Tasker at HMP Leeds; Julie Norman; Adrian Lay; Chris Carlisle for our wonderful website.

Molly-Ann, and the many children whom we have had the pleasure of meeting over the past few years, also the little angels Jack and Nisa, who are no longer with us, thank you all, for your contribution to our story. Your fight and determination has enriched us.

'Dr Mike' – you never leave a stone unturned and always listen to our comments and fears; Helen Greenwood, who is always only a phone call away.

Alice has asked that we thank two special people, nurse Rachael from Dewsbury District Hospital and play therapist Carol Simpson. Alice has grown to trust you both every step of the way in her young, at times troubled, but eternally inspirational life.

Finally, we give thanks and praise to God for His love, strength and guidance.

Dean and Carol Maddocks

Thanks to Ian Dick, Douglas Moulding, Richard Frederiks, Kathy Fletcher, John Howard, David Berry, Sean and Mandy Kenyon, Lesley Wordsworth, Sam and Virginia Sherbourne, Nance Parry, Anne Lloyd, Jane Donovan, Alison Leach, Sharon Benjamin, Richard Mason, Melanie Letts, Bob Crocker, Jeremy Robson, Rob Dimery, Shirley Cummings, Carolyn Desourdy, Peter Brown and Alan Green.

Malcolm Stacey

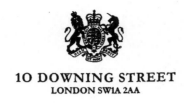

1O DOWNING STREET
LONDON SW1A 2AA

THE PRIME MINISTER

Anyone who meets Alice or her parents comes away with tremendous admiration for them, together with a desire to do all you can to help.

Alice is a lovely, lively, courageous child. I still keep on my desk the 'worry dolls' which she made and gave me when she visited No 10.

In their own way, Dean and Carol are equally remarkable. The news that your child is seriously ill is something that every parent dreads. Faced with the enormous pressures such a blow must place on any family, it must be easy to hide away.

But Dean and Carol have shown astonishing energy and commitment not just to help their own daughter but all those who need bone marrow transplants.

Their efforts, and those of other families, have done a huge amount to focus attention on the need for more bone marrow donors. It's no exaggeration to say that these efforts will save scores of lives.

Tony Blair

March 2003

Alice's Story

Hi, I'm Alice. I am 10yrs old. I live with my mum Carol, dad Dean, big sister Chloe and not forgetting my dog Charlie.
We live in a town called Dewsbury.

I have an illness called Aplastic Anaemia. This means my bone marrow is not working properly. I was 7yrs old when I found out. I did not really understand what it was all about. Mum and Dad tried to explain it to me but I never thought it was anything to worry about. And any way I felt fine!

Before I was poorly, I enjoyed swimming, Dancing, bike riding and spending time with my friends. They are Abi, Lyidia, Amelia, Fay, Olivia, Sarah, Tuscany, Lucy, and Natalie.

Because of my illness I have spent many weeks at St James's Hospital in Leeds. This was a long time to be away from home, but my Mum and Dad stayed with me all the time. Chloe often came to visit. Some of the treatment made me very poorly, I don't like to look back and remember it because it makes me feel sad.

For the past 3yrs Dr Mike and some other doctors have been trying to find a special person who has the same bone marrow as me. They have not found any one yet. Mum tells me I have a special bone marrow that not very many people have. So the search goes on.........

People say I am brave but I think my sister Chloe is also brave because she had to spend lots of time away from me and my mum and dad. She had to stay with my grandma and Granddad or with friends of our family. Chloe sometimes felt sad about this, she just wanted us all to be home together. Chloe was also very brave when she had to give the Doctors some of her blood to see if her bone marrow was the same as mine. We had to wait a few weeks before the test came back we then found out that Chloe's bone marrow was different.

I have had to have lots of blood transfusions over the past few years. I think the people who give blood are very kind. They help to save people's lives, just like people who give bone marrow.

Since I became ill I have met some very nice people and done things I may not have done if I had not been poorly. I went with Dad to watch Man United and we met some of the players. My favorite player is Ryan Giggs. I have also met Prince Charles, Liz Dawn, Chris Chittle, the cast from "EMMERDALE", Kazia Pelkia, S Club Seven, Nicki Chapmen and Gareth Gates.

I have also done something very special. I went To Number 10 Downing Street for tea with The Prime Minister Tony Blair, Cherie Blair and their baby Leo. He is lovely. I was very excited. Inside it was beautiful, like a mansion, everyone made us feel very special.

I hope you enjoy reading our story.

Alice
x

Love, Alice. x

Introduction

A pretty blue-and-green ball, surrounded by nothing, spins in black space. Earth – our planet, encircled by the delicate tracery of vapour trails from constantly moving metallic shapes that leap continents and oceans and time zones. One such silvery marvel soars up from the Leeds–Bradford airport and steadily purrs along in search of holiday sun. The few passengers who look down see a spider's web of street lighting marking a cluster of towns to the south of Leeds: Dewsbury, Hanging Heaton, Heckmondwike, Ossett and Batley. Like all communities seen from the air, the streets far below seem insubstantial. But every family in these neat houses has a tale to tell. The most remarkable of these stories – one which people find hard to believe is true – comes from a small 1930s semidetached in Hanging Heaton. The Maddocks family live here. Dean, the wavy-haired, good-looking father, is a constable in the West Yorkshire Police force. Quiet, sensible, well mannered, he's a far cry from the bombastic, bitter coppers projected by writers of hackneyed screenplays. His wife Carol, brown-eyed and vibrant, is a social worker. She's more extrovert and outspoken than her husband, but not in a brash, showy way. They have two children, twelve-year-old Chloe and Alice, who's ten. They had one simple aim above all else – to be happy – and they were. Very happy. Until one day when an ugly catastrophe toppled from a cloudless sky...

They were told that Alice only had a short time to live.

What is the worst thing that could happen to you? What if it suddenly came about? What if a doctor broke it to you that your child had a rare disease that threatened his or her life? What would you do? Have you thought about it? Of course you have. We all have. Most parents would trustingly put their unenviable destiny in the hands of a hospital consultant – and do nothing else. A few might go a little further and leave a few collecting boxes on shop counters so as to send their child to Florida on holiday.

The Maddocks family took a different course. They refused to meekly accept what was happening to their younger daughter. They decided to put up a fight. And what a tussle it turned out to be! An almighty battle with authority, which has projected them into the very heart of British politics.

As a broadcaster who's made a good living out of covering the awful setbacks of families in trouble, I am now doing a bit of voluntary work – agitating for children who are up against it. Guilt, I suppose – for a wasted life. One night at the beginning of February 2001, Dean Maddocks rang my home. His request was put quietly, without emotion. He's that sort of man. He would understand if I turned him down, but would I help get some publicity for Alice? His hope was that if ordinary people were told of his daughter's plight, they would sign up to give bone marrow. And if just one donor could be found with the right match, then Alice would have a future.

As it was, I never needed to work very hard for Dean and Carol. They quickly surpassed my poor skills at manipulating the Establishment. They learned to run rings round doctors, medical administrators, politicians, television moguls and crafty denizens of the British press. Soon they made luminaries, people at the pinnacle of the National Blood Service, think seriously about what they were doing – and they changed government policy forever.

But this isn't just a story of pushing people at the top. It's a tale of the terrific love that binds a family in trouble; of Alice having to endure agony and indignity in hospital; of the tragic mites living out their last days prematurely in beds around her; and of those who turned their backs on or tried to exploit the family's torment. For if this is a tale which teases out the best in people, it also brings out the worst.

This is a story of our times. It *has* to be told. And I feel privileged in being able to record the astounding chronicle of the remarkable Alice Maddocks in these pages.

Malcolm Stacey
March 2003

PART ONE

A Fall in the Garden

The small grey town of Batley is still best known to the outside world for once having been the unlikely setting for performances by legendary stars of show business. Such internationally acclaimed artistes as Shirley Bassey, Louis Armstrong, Tony Bennett, Roy Orbison, Tony Hancock and Sammy Davis Junior topped the bill at the Batley Variety Club, now a disco club. But on a cold winter's night at the end of 2001, it was a little girl who stole the limelight in this town. Pushing down the huge horizontal bar on top of a red box, tiny Alice Maddocks, her pretty olive skin pink with excitement, switched on the town's Christmas lights. The cheers and clapping went on and on.

Alice is a local celebrity, a real draw. People in Yorkshire read more about her and think more about her than any of the show biz stars named above. She means more to the retired miners, mill workers, dustmen, solicitors, teachers, hairdressers, teenagers and pensioners here than anybody in the tinsel world. She's won awards as a 'young achiever', her teachers idolise her, youngsters beg for autographs. But hers is a celebrity not conceived by material success or achievement. Hers is an unwanted celebrity born of courage. Every day Alice fights for her life. Her deeply impressive struggle has won many hearts, first of friends and neighbours and then of the nation at large.

Her story is astounding, involving some of the best-known people in the land. Her campaign to win back her health has brought about astonishing results in the world of politics. Yet her life is still in the balance. And every day, that struggle for existence becomes more desperate. The time when everyone in her family was completely

3

free of health problems, any problems at all actually, now seems a long time ago. Though it isn't...

                                    * * *

In May 2000, eighteen months before Alice switched on the Christmas lights in the town of Batley, her parents, Carol and Dean, went to bed one night in their neat and comfortable home. Nothing was preying on her mind but Carol's sleep was disturbed by a terrible dream. Her mother Pat, whom she idolised, had died suddenly of a brain haemorrhage at the early age of 58, some six years before, while in prayer at her bedside. Carol had never dreamed about her mother until that night.

Pat's mother was also present in the short but chilling dream. Carol had frequently pictured her grandmother since her death sixteen years previously, but she had always seemed joyful, never without her lovely smile. In the dream the smile was missing. Gran was sitting in an armchair, leaning slightly forward, looking grim and tense. There was no sign of the living room where the chair used to be. The chair seemed suspended in darkness, moving slightly as if in a wind. Carol's mother hovered behind Gran, watching over her shoulder. Both women were talking simultaneously, their words inaudible. The atmosphere was gloomy, oppressive and filled with foreboding.

Carol was shaken by the vividness of the scene, which spilled over with detail, in fierce colour. 'Both Mum and Gran had this sad expression on their faces. You know, extremely woeful. They stared at me with mournful eyes, obviously perturbed that I couldn't understand. Were they cross with me? Or perhaps it was pity. Anyway, it was awful.'

Carol still shudders when she recalls this eerie dream. 'I wondered what it was all about and thought they were trying to give me a warning of some kind. But what was it? Both of them were from previous generations, so I wondered afterwards if they were saying something awful about the next generation – our two lovely girls, Chloe and Alice. I was really scared.' Dean told her not to be silly.

The next evening, one of Carol's favourite TV series, *Peak Practice*, introduced a story line about a little girl with leukaemia. Carol, deeply moved, turned to her husband. 'I hope we never have

to face that. How do real families cope with anything so awful?'
Sadly, they were soon to learn.

* * *

A few weeks later, in May 2000, Chloe, a quiet, affectionate girl
aged eleven, pointed out her younger sister's legs were newly-
covered with what seemed to be freckles. They didn't tell their
mother. But a day or two later, while soaping Alice in the bath, Carol
noticed the tiny marks, too. By now they looked more like bruises
than freckles and were no longer confined to her legs, but had
spread all over her body. Carol had no idea what the tiny blemishes
were, but didn't the little girl in *Peak Practice* have the same kind
of marks on her arms?

Dismissing the thought as 'paranoid', Carol forgot about the
strange spots. But they soon drifted back into her mind. A small
voice in her head told her there was something 'not quite right'
about Alice. 'It was a spooky feeling that wouldn't go away. I
couldn't put my finger on it. She didn't seem ill in any way. She was
as happy as ever. She didn't even look pale. She was full of her
usual energy. But something unseen was wrong. I wasn't happy
about her.'

Yet life at home went on as normal. Carol continued to counsel
abused and neglected children in the care of the local authority.
Dean worked in and around Bradford police station. The two girls
went, with their usual merry enthusiasm, to the friendly village
school in Hanging Heaton.

The next Friday, after school, all the family crowded into their
diminutive bathroom to get ready for a 'fun evening' in the church
hall. The two girls were splashing in the bath together, fighting for
the soap, when Chloe asked, 'Mummy, have you seen how many
bruises Alice's got? I've just counted them. There are eighteen.'

Carol moved up to peer at Alice's leg. She chided her older
daughter. 'Don't be silly, Chloe. Just get yourself washed. We'll be
late for all the games.'

For three members of the family, it was a lovely night out. The
girls and Dean revelled in musical chairs, pass the parcel and a bit
of disco dancing. But Carol seemed distracted and glum. She was

becoming more anxious about Alice. As she told Dean later, 'I didn't want to hear about those damn bruises from Chloe. I just wanted to gag her. I knew exactly how many spots Alice has on her body. I've been counting them as they come – one by one.'

But Carol and Dean still shirked the problem of those ominous spots. They kidded themselves that the small purple marks were the result of rough games in the playground. They continued to believe this though the marks were now spreading fast. They were no longer confined to Alice's arms and legs, but were encroaching on her stomach and back.

* * *

Later, Carol couldn't understand why they didn't take Alice to the doctor as soon as the marks were discovered. 'We had a child with a body covered in bruises, and we pushed it aside and did nothing. It seems irresponsible now, but deep down, I suppose we must have been afraid to learn what they were.'

Dean shares the guilt. 'We'd been blessed with brilliant health. The awful possibility that Alice was seriously ill with something we didn't recognise, not like a cold or a stomach upset, was a possibility we didn't think we could handle.'

Soon afterwards, their friend Caroline's little girl celebrated her first communion service at the local church. The Maddocks family followed them to their home for a small party in the sunny garden. But what was a happy occasion took a frightening turn when Alice stumbled on the grass. She cut her right knee. Carol heard her daughter crying and rushed to help. She was glad to see it was only a slight cut, not half an inch long and not all that deep. She dabbed at it with a tissue. But the small trickle of blood wouldn't stop. It continued to drip down into the grass. Carol asked Caroline for a plaster. But the blood soaked through the dressing, and still kept oozing out. It was ten minutes before the thin red flow dried up.

Dean asked Caroline for advice. She was a nurse who'd worked with children. 'What do you think it could be?' he asked anxiously. He also decided it was high time to break his personal taboo and mention those spots. 'Caroline, we've noticed that Alice has bruises spreading all over her body. And if you look closely, you'll see some tiny purple dots on her face, too.'

Caroline was reassuring. 'Oh, I wouldn't worry about that. Just take her to the health centre. She's probably got a fairly harmless virus.'

But Dean guessed that Caroline, out of kindness, was holding something back. Surely, she would have come across such conspicuous symptoms many times during twenty years' working with sick children. She must know a lot more about this than she was letting on. So why was she so vague? He'd never seen anything like these marks before, and he suspected they did not signify any trivial childhood ailment. Apart from the bruises and purple spots, their daughter now had a tiny cut that wouldn't stop bleeding.

Carol believed that her friend was secretly concerned, and pressed her for a few more possible explanations. But if Caroline was worried, she didn't show it. She repeated that they should take Alice to the health centre. But by now the Maddocks were quietly concerned and made a doctor's appointment for the next afternoon.

The Yellow Post-It Note

Alice went to school as usual in the morning, while Carol wondered what she would say to the doctor. 'Apart from these bruises, Alice is perfectly fit,' she confided to Dean. 'There's no pain, no sore throat, no temperature, nothing. Alice has always been such a healthy child, and she's certainly in the pink just now.'

At the surgery, the doctor commented that it was four years since Alice had last visited him. He examined the bruises on her legs, chest and face. Carol and Dean nervously searched his face for a reaction, either of relief or trepidation, but found only professional calm. Something seemed to be wrong, though, because, still with a poker face, he rang the district hospital in Dewsbury and arranged for Alice to give a blood sample. It must be done that day, he insisted. Though trying to stay calm, Carol was extremely worried by the doctor's controlled urgency. 'My mind was racing, palms sweating and I had an overwhelming urge to be sick. What was going on? He wanted Alice to provide a blood sample quickly and insisted on the results the next day. The urgency of it all scared me.'

Dean recollects, 'I tried to tell myself this was no big deal. I didn't really believe it. Even so, we stayed cheerful because we didn't want to worry Alice.' A thought raced through Carol's mind that the results of blood tests often took at least a week to come through. Why was the doctor hurrying things along?

Mother and daughter went to the nearby Dewsbury District Hospital. Although Alice had never been inside a hospital before, she was chatty and cheerful as a phial of blood was drawn from her arm. The nurse was surprised she didn't flinch when the needle punctured the skin. This was the first time Carol found herself impressed by her daughter's casual reaction to medical treatment. But it was only the beginning. Alice's courage would be something to marvel at again and again. But at the time Carol wondered if this first blood test was really necessary. 'To see nurses scurrying round us, surrounded by scary equipment, white walls and that peculiar hospital smell was very upsetting for Alice and I wondered what we were doing there.' Once again, she tried to push Alice's dramatic but painless symptoms to the back of her brain.

* * *

It was early next morning that Carol and Alice returned with Dean to the doctor's surgery. By now, Carol had convinced herself that the blood test was only a precaution: that Alice was so obviously healthy that no serious ailment could possibly threaten her. Doctors had to be really careful these days because of those patients who sued at the slightest mistake. Perhaps that new greedy trend had led their GP into being a bit too cautious.

The little girl beside her interrupted these thoughts. Alice was grumbling about her second visit to the surgery in two days. She wanted to be back in school and was fretting about missing her lunchtime chat with friends. All three went into the doctor's room. Carol idly noticed a yellow post-it note stuck to a folder on a desk. 'I knew I had no right to read it. It was quite obviously private but I couldn't help myself. I read the three words and it turned my blood cold...

- Alice Maddocks - Leukaemia?

'It was just like somebody had pulled a curtain down on our lives. I felt sick and empty inside,' she remembers vividly. 'I wanted to cry. I had a sense of disbelief. Only a few hours before I'd dropped her off at school as a normal and healthy seven-year-old. Now, I was being told she had a life-threatening disease. I felt numb and blank. My head was pounding, as if it had been hit with a sledge hammer. I just wanted to sob my heart out but I knew I couldn't because it would frighten Alice. And all this happened before we even spoke to the doctor – we had this awful, awful news on a tiny note written by goodness knows who. I was convinced it couldn't be anything serious because she was looking so well. I felt like just running away, a massive desire to escape from this doctor's surgery.'

Carol mentally rattled off some grim portents of the future. All her hopes of a happy and productive life were melting away and she wasn't aware of the doctor entering the room. But she dimly heard him say gently, 'I fear Alice may have something quite seriously wrong with her.'

This was too much to take in. Dean felt he was in a film where an actor playing a doctor was speaking to a different couple in slow motion. What was he saying now? They must try and concentrate. The doctor seemed to want Alice to go back to hospital for more tests. Carol swallowed and somehow managed to muster the courage to ask, 'Are you trying to tell me that our daughter has leukaemia?' She knew that Alice, who was sitting unconcernedly between them, wouldn't understand the question.

'Yes,' he replied very gently, 'I'm sorry, but I am.'

The couple turned and looked fearfully at each other. Their expressions betrayed shocked disbelief. Their beautiful, healthy, clever, carefree daughter was stricken with a life-threatening disease which everyone dreads. Tests would be needed to confirm it, of course, but the doctor seemed pretty sure. As a policeman, Dean is used to giving sad news to others, often to parents. But he wasn't ready for this. His mind went numb and so did Carol's. They can't remember how they reached their car without scaring Alice, but doubted that they succeeded.

They didn't go straight to the hospital for the new tests ordered by their doctor. Instead, they drove to the home of Carol's sister, Sue Dymond and her husband, Richard. They needed someone to talk to, to help them gather their thoughts and overcome the cold panic in their hearts. Their relatives were as sympathetic and reassuring as they could be in such ghastly circumstances, but it was difficult to think of anything comforting to say. A cup of coffee helped a little and the Maddocks finally set off to Dewsbury District Hospital.

'It was an awful journey into the unknown,' said Carol. 'We had no idea what to expect, other than we would probably get confirmation that Alice's life was threatened by a dreadful disease.' As they drove on grimly, Alice talked only about her school lunch, asking over and over again, 'I'm not going to miss it, am I, Mummy?' Neither parent could tear themselves away from their gloomy thoughts to answer.

A specialist nurse met the family at the hospital gates. From that moment, Helen Greenwood, cheerful and understanding, was to play an important role in Alice's life. She proved to be someone the family could confide in and who always strove to put them at ease. She led them all into a large waiting room that was both modern and clean. Cancer patients populated it. Alice was the only child there.

'I took one look at these poor people, and Dean did, and so did Alice. And the fear in Alice's eyes was awful to see,' Carol recalls, sadly. 'This wasn't part of our world at all! These folks were having chemotherapy, and though it doesn't seem very nice to say so, Alice was frightened by them. Many of them had no hair and we could see she was disturbed by this. Everyone was kind and friendly, but even that didn't help. We couldn't raise our spirits to smile back.'

Dean tried to explain to Alice that the baldness wasn't permanent, that it was only part of the treatment. But explaining that to a tearful, alarmed seven-year-old was difficult. The couple felt helpless. They couldn't imagine the effect of that group of patients on the mind of a child who, until the previous day, had never even seen the inside of a hospital.

(Many of the patients the Maddocks met that day are now in remission and look a picture of health. Others who're still under treatment in the clinic have since become 'special friends' of Alice.)

A New Hope

Alice had a series of tests on her first visit to the district hospital and the results showed her blood was short of platelets. These tiny components of blood, formed in bone marrow, help to cause clotting. Without them it is possible to bleed to death. But at that time Dean and Carol had no idea what they were. Helen Greenwood led Alice away to draw pictures, while a kindly specialist in her mid-forties, Dr Mary Chapple, spelled out the results. Carol could have hugged her. She gave them a shred of hope.

She said Alice could have leukaemia or a total failure of the bone marrow. But there was a third possibility – a virus that had temporarily attacked the immune system. Dean remembers how much happier they both were when Dr Chapple conceded that she didn't think it was bone marrow failure because that was so rare, and that the most likely explanation was a virus, from which Alice would make a spontaneous recovery.

The couple thought that such a bug sounded pretty plausible. Didn't their friend Caroline say that a 'harmless virus' had probably caused the mysterious bruising and purple spots? Perhaps everything was going to be all right, after all. They agreed to return the next day for Alice to have a 'bone marrow biopsy'. This sounded difficult and it is. Not only would surgeons take a sample of bone marrow from inside Alice's hip, they would also remove a piece of bone. This would later be dissected in a laboratory, to allow experts to examine every minute layer of its structure. Only then could the boffins tell what was happening to stop Alice's bone marrow from producing blood cells.

* * *

Because of the family's natural alarm at this prospect, Dean's mother was recruited for moral support. Seven years earlier, Joan Maddocks had watched Alice's birth, and they now enjoyed a close relationship. As Alice was about to have her first operation, it was going to be up to Joan to calm her. 'You're going to sleep for a short while, so there's nothing to worry about,' she said softly. Under house rules, only one parent was allowed to watch a child go under an anaesthetic. It was agreed that Dean should go into the theatre, leaving Carol and Joan to worry outside the rubber-edged double doors.

Carol was secretly relieved by the 'one-parent-only' dictum; she couldn't bring herself to watch Alice slipping under. 'I was a coward. I couldn't go in. I wanted Dean to do it.' She was also troubled by another anxiety. 'I had this strange fear they would take Alice into the theatre, put her to sleep, and I would never see her again.'

Alice, however, was concerned about something else. She was hungry and kept asking for her favourite snack, 'When am I going to get a corned beef sandwich?' With a reassuring wink at his wife, Dean delicately took Alice's hand and they disappeared inside the theatre, where someone pricked Alice's tiny palm with a syringe of anaesthetic. After five minutes, Dean came back alone. He'd been crying. 'In all our then twelve years together, I had never seen Dean cry before. He is not that type, not one to show his emotions, but he looked frightened to death. His shoulders were slumped. He looked like a broken man. I thought now she's asleep, at last I can show my feelings of relief without letting her know there was anything serious to worry about.

'We were standing in the corridor and Dean walked over to me. We clung to each other tightly and wept. We were so desperately afraid for the future,' Carol explained. Half an hour later, Carol,

Dean and Joan were gathered round a child's bed, waiting for Alice to come round. 'She was in a green rubbery hospital gown, so small, so vulnerable, sleeping so peacefully,' Carol recalls fondly. 'There wasn't a trace of worry on her face. It was a magic moment to see our daughter looking so serene and innocent. Yet all three of us knew in our hearts there were dreadful things in her future. Awful, unspeakable things.'

Both parents had been told everything hinged on how many platelets Alice's bone marrow could produce. If the tally was high, there was little to worry about; Alice would probably soon recover. Helen Greenwood had been working with the surgeons who carried out the biopsy, and must have known by then how healthy Alice's platelet count was. She joined them around the bed as Alice continued to sleep. Yet neither Dean nor Carol could bring themselves to ask the crucial question. Granny Maddocks was braver. 'What's the normal platelet count?' she inquired quietly.

'About 280.'

'And Alice's?'

'Twenty-two.'

Everybody reeled with shock. It seemed that Alice's fate had been sealed. She must be very ill indeed. They wondered how her body could function at all with such an abnormally low count. But Alice was stirring in bed. And her parents and grandmother forced themselves to cheer up. 'Now can I have my corned beef sandwich?' she asked. Everyone laughed. Carol wanted to wrap up her daughter in cotton wool, sneak out of the hospital and drive her safely home. Alice, though, had other ideas. And in less than an hour, their book-loving daughter was back at school.

* * *

The family were told to expect the full results of the bone marrow biopsy on the Friday, two days after the operation. Carol couldn't sleep on the Thursday night. Her head was in turmoil, with fragments of gloomy thoughts slipping in and out of her mind. In the early hours she gave up the struggle. She dressed and crept downstairs. She sat on the lounge sofa, the light from a street lamp falling on her face. Her eyes closed.

'I prayed to God that He wouldn't take our little girl from us. I asked that her biopsy would not show anything to worry about. But more than that, I prayed He would give us the strength and courage to deal with everything that lay ahead.' She was still for a long time, repeating her silent plea to the Almighty over and over as the yellow of the street lamp outside gradually yielded to a shy grey dawn. Then suddenly her mood changed. The prayers ceased. 'I began to feel quite angry with God, wondering about my faith. Was it worth anything, now? What was it all about, anyway? What had we done to have this terrible trouble thrown at us?' And even harder to explain, 'What had an innocent girl done to deserve the kind of suffering that surely lies ahead?'

Carol began to sob, dabbing at her pale cheeks with a tissue. Calmer now, but making no attempt to staunch her tears, she reflected, 'It must be part of some divine plan; God knows best.' She continued to weep alone while Dean slept. On and off the tears came, as the morning light gathered strength. The girls also slumbered deeply, oblivious to Carol's all-night vigil and crushing anxieties.

In the morning, back in Dewsbury District Hospital, Carol and Dean felt layers of anxiety fall away. The results of the biopsy showed Alice did not have leukaemia. This all-too-common blood disease is what the Maddocks feared more than any other illness. All parents dread it. So that was OK then. But if not leukaemia, what did Alice have that caused the purple bruises and the failure of her blood to clot properly? Dr Chapple explained to the couple that there was an unidentified abnormality in Alice's bone marrow and that she would have to be monitored for a week or so. But at least leukaemia had been ruled out. And when the couple returned home in a buoyant mood, they genuinely believed they had agonised all week over nothing. As she entered the house, Carol started to sob. Chloe asked, 'What's the matter, Mum?' Alice hugged her mother in alarm.

Her father explained to Alice that grown-ups sometimes cried with joy. 'I told her Mummy was crying because everything was going to be all right. She hadn't got the nasty disease we thought she had and she was well again. Later, we bitterly regretted telling Alice there was nothing to worry about. The worst thing we thought she faced was leukaemia so when they said she didn't have it, we thought she was safe and would soon be well, and she probably only had a virus. But when we were told differently and that she had a much more rare condition, we were sorry we'd given our daughter false hopes.'

The as-yet-unspecified abnormality in Alice's bone marrow was caused by a sinister and rare condition, even more deadly than leukaemia. And that disease could only get worse.

* * *

But for the time being, family life went on as usual. Alice seemed fit and well. Her appetite grew. She was energetic, boisterous, enthusiastic. She continued to blossom at school. She played and laughed with Chloe and her friends. She also went to hospital once or twice 'to be monitored'. But the doctors were talking a different language, seemingly from a science fiction novel. It was all about platelets, neutrophils (white blood cells) and haemoglobin. Dean and Carol, understanding none of this and not caring either, were confident that Alice's condition had been little more than an unpleasant scare.

But on 16 June 2000, something happened that changed the family's life for ever. Alice fell in the school playground. Her nose was cut and bruised and she developed two big black eyes, made darker and wider by the dearth of platelets in her blood. Once again, the blood was hard to staunch. To make things worse, Carol and Dean were out shopping at home when the tumble occurred. They returned home at lunchtime to find an alarming message on the answerphone. The teacher who called said that Alice had been rushed to hospital for an emergency blood transfusion.

Carol was horrified. She'd read that blood products could be tainted by AIDS or hepatitis B, and was unaware that a foolproof screening operation was now in place. Later in hospital, Carol looked at the bag feeding a stranger's blood into her daughter's arm, and her alarm was replaced by a surge of pure gratitude. 'I longed to thank the donor in person. It seemed such a perfect thing to have done.' That sense of gratefulness was to grow even stronger over the months, because from then on, the Maddocks family was to rely on hundreds of donors just to keep Alice alive.

After her fall at school, Alice began going to hospital twice a week to see Dr Chapple, who would test for platelets in her blood. After one such test, she later rang the Maddocks' home one evening with harsh news. She was concerned. Alice's platelet count was now exceptionally low. She explained she was passing the case to a specialist on children's blood diseases at St James's, the vast Leeds hospital made famous by the fly-on-the wall television programme, *Jimmy's*. Carol and Dean were startled by the call. 'We feared Alice's condition must be getting serious now, possibly dangerous. Why else would a busy consultant make an evening call to our house? Still no firm diagnosis had been given, so it was with cold dread that I asked Dr Chapple what she thought the problem might be,' Carol recalled.

The doctor said she was not sure but it was possibly one of two different conditions. Both ailments were life-threatening, though Dr Chapple drew back from saying this. She thought that Alice had either aplastic anaemia or myelodysplasia. Carol, who took the call, felt a sharp barb of fear. But Dr Chapple said that although some of Alice's red cells were showing signs of change, not enough altered cells had been found to make myelodysplasia the certain diagnosis. Aplastic anaemia was just as likely to be the cause. Carol and Dean were to discover later that a severe form of aplastic anaemia was really the correct choice. But just then they were ignorant of both conditions.

Hearing both possible illnesses given a name somehow brought succour to Carol. 'It just didn't sound too serious. We knew that leukaemia, which everybody knows is dangerous, had been ruled out. So I thought there'd be quick and easy treatments for both these unfamiliar conditions – and that Alice would soon be her old self again.' She phoned her brother-in-law Richard and asked him to check the Internet for the most likely of the two conditions – aplastic anaemia. He rang back and told lies. 'Nothing much to worry about,' he said casually. He was glad Carol couldn't see him shaking. What he'd seen on his home computer frightened him. He couldn't bring himself to tell Carol or Dean the grim, desolate details he'd picked from the screen. If Alice had this disease, she could be in real danger. Mortal danger.

* * *

Alice continued to have transfusions in hospital, until towards the end of June when a routine donation of blood made her ill. Her tongue and lips swelled up. Her face became bloated. Her eyes took on an Oriental aspect. These were classic symptoms of an allergic reaction. Nurses hurriedly gave anti-histamines to quell what they recognised as the body's hostile response to the foreign platelets. Thankfully, the symptoms subsided, though not altogether.

Alice could have stayed in hospital until she'd fully recovered, but Carol took her home to bed. She was unwell for the rest of the day, but with typical fighting spirit, pestered her mother to allow her to get up the next day for a friend's birthday party. 'I watched her intently and felt heavy-hearted at how my daughter, so carefree and healthy only two weeks ago, now seemed pale, drawn and delicate. She was wilting under the strain of so many blood transfusions. I remember looking at her ears and they were almost transparent because she was starting to be so anaemic. I felt so apart from everyone else at the party.'

Sadly, Alice was now feeling unwell for most of the time. The family entered a dark unhappy tunnel. The demands of their jobs began to weigh on both parents. Dean, the highest earner, continued to work in Bradford's car crime unit, supported by understanding colleagues and superiors. But Carol, who's part of a team looking after young people in council care, took two weeks off. Despite feeling she'd let her young people down, she was naturally more concerned by Alice's worsening condition. The little girl's latest tests showed her platelet count was still dropping. It was soon down to a lowly nineteen – less than a tenth of what it should be. And this was only three days after she'd had an urgent platelet transfusion. Her parents were appalled by the news, but tried as usual to be cheerful in front of the children.

With the platelet count now so low, the transfer of responsibility for Alice from Dewsbury District Hospital to St James's in Leeds had to be arranged quickly. For Alice, Chloe and their parents, the strain of hospital life was only just beginning...

St Jimmy's

The family's first visit to St James's was to the Children's Day Hospital, a two-storey detached building, painted pink. They found a huge playroom-cum-waiting room, which had been given, in honour of the season, a summer holiday theme. The walls were arrayed with bright paintings of buckets and spades and sandcastles executed by the young patients. Dean and Carol suspected some of these junior artists might no longer be able to hold a brush, and they were saddened by their beautiful work, rather than cheered. These bright pictures did little to hide the dilapidated nature of the Day Hospital. Dean, a keen amateur decorator, noticed stained cracks in the plaster where water had seeped in. The paint on the woodwork was dingy and chipped. Doors didn't open without a struggle. Windows were opaque with grime.

There were other problems, too. Babies were lumped in the playroom with self-conscious youngsters in their teens. Dean's first thought was that this was no place for kids in pain, undergoing treatments that could make them feel even more ill than before. There was no comfort here, either physical or mental. The huge room presented a noisy scene of seeming chaos where privacy didn't exist. They found themselves surrounded by the rattle and clatter of, among other things, televisions, Play Station consoles, toy drums and children careering round in pedal cars. And mixed in with that racket were the occasional screams of youngsters in fear or pain, or just gently sobbing.

All around them were the blank faces of adults trying to keep hopelessness out of their expressions. They were too unhappy to talk to each other. Occasionally, some parents received a diagnosis for the first time; a few had good news, and others did not. There was no absence of worry and dread in here.

At the Dewsbury hospital clinic, Alice's fellow-patients had been mainly adults. Mentally, Carol put Alice in a different, safer category to them. Alice was a child. She did not have cancer. Therefore she was not in danger. But in this broad room at St James's there were no grown-ups. Alice couldn't be singled out as somehow being above serious illness. She was just like them, a child with a grave disease. There were tiny babies, toddlers children and teenagers, all in various stages of treatment, chemotherapy and radiotherapy. Some of these young patients were evidently in a wretched state.

Carol strained not to be visibly shocked by this desperately sad room, but she was profoundly disturbed nonetheless. So was Alice. A row of grown-ups, totally bald due to the temporary side effects of chemotherapy, is one thing. But to see patients of her own age and even younger without hair, when she's so proud of her own long thick locks, made Alice very uneasy. Wriggling in her seat, not knowing what to do with her hands, she couldn't sit still. She kept asking to go home.

After an hour, the three of them were called to see a man they'd often heard mentioned and praised – St James's children's blood specialist, Dr Mike Richards. He was known around the hospital as 'Dr Mike'. Carol's first thought was that he was too young for his job – possibly in his mid-thirties. He was a tall, smartly dressed man but not in a stiff or starchy way. Dean noticed a rather nervous, diffident manner. He seemed hesitant, afraid of offending.

Carol was also sizing up Alice's new consultant. She would have preferred a silver-haired medic in his sixties, someone with years of experience, a seasoned specialist who would not like to be called 'Dr Mike'. Could she really trust her daughter's life to such young hands? He looked, wrongly as they discovered, not long out of medical school. What rare qualities had he had time to develop, she wondered? But she cheered up when he spoke. He was able to explain what he thought was happening to Alice in a warm, clear and jargon-free way. They were reassured that he didn't seem at all worried or overwhelmed by Alice's case. Even so, the couple were rather perturbed when he asked for another bone marrow biopsy the very next day. They'd been hoping – not very rationally – that Alice would be 'signed off'.

'Dr Mike' asked Alice if another biopsy would be all right with her? 'Yes,' she said nonchalantly, 'that will be fine.'

* * *

The family returned to St James's at 8.30 a.m. Alice was cheerful, clutching Lady, her cuddly toy King Charles spaniel. 'She was her jolly little self,' recalled Carol, 'until we entered that room again, with all those poor children. Then she suddenly became anxious. She was even more upset when she heard that she would soon be sent to sleep for another operation. It was disconcerting for us, but so much more terrifying for her.'

Her parents, smiling, but inwardly sagging with worry, promised to be waiting when she came round. This time Carol did not stay on the other side of the swing doors. There was no excuse anyway because in this hospital there was no 'one-parent-only' rule. All three went hand-in-hand into the small operating theatre.

'I knew I had to be strong this time. I realised it wasn't fair on Dean to take the whole responsibility,' Carol elucidated. 'We both knew we were going to carry this burden together, come what may, until Alice recovered.'

A cheery nurse distracted Alice with a teddy bear while the anaesthetist secretly pricked her hand. Her eyes rolled and she was asleep in seconds. The old fear returned. Carol dreaded tearfully that her darling would never wake up, given her frail state, her weakened blood supply. Soon, placid capable surgeons sucked more bone marrow from her slender pelvis, while the couple waited outside, their foreheads damp, their hands clenched. It was over quickly. Afterwards back on the ward, with hearts beating quickly, two anxious sets of eyes peered down at Alice waiting for her to recover consciousness. They were rewarded with 'when do I get my corned beef sandwich?' Once again they were astonished at how quickly Alice became her normal rather pushy self again.

'I have to go back to school this afternoon, Mummy,' she said urgently. Carol remembered the end-of-term concert was that day. But now it was out of the question. 'No, Alice, I'm sorry. But you've just had an operation – and you're certainly not well enough to do that!'

'I am. I'm all right.'

'You're definitely not, Alice.'

'I am.'

The to-ing and fro-ing continued for a bit until Alice got her way. She often did in those early days. Both parents tried not to give in to their daughter's every wish of course, but it was a skill they only mastered later on. Anyway, Carol was proud of her daughter's persistence (she preferred not to call it obstinacy). Alice intended to be in the play, and no silly illness was going to stop her. It was a tale set in a toy factory and she played an elf. 'She had a beaming smile when she was on stage. But I could see her eyes looking heavy and her skin had that waxy, transparent look. As we sat watching her pretending to sew toys on the elves' factory line, my mind kept wondering, "Will this be the last school play we'll see her in? Will she be there at Christmas?" I was looking into the future but in a negative way. Part of me thought if I think like that, the worst picture, then it won't happen and only the opposite will come true and Alice will be OK. We were so proud of her that day but much later, looking at school photographs of that summer term show, Dean remarked that Alice looked dreadful. She seemed chalky white, so tottery and vulnerable, about to topple over.' But Dean added with satisfaction, 'She had a terrific smile on her face and it was there on every picture. Though she must have been feeling terrible, she gave it her all and was the best elf in Dewsbury that day!'

'The Man's Talking Rubbish...'

When mother, father and daughter went back to St James's in July 2000 for the results of the latest biopsy, they found the clinic was even busier than before. 'It was absolutely heaving with children,' said Carol. 'Older children and tiny mites were on drips, having blood transfusions, food infusions, chemotherapy, all sorts. Some had tubes coming from their tiny bodies. Many were lying down, worn out by what they were going through.' Yet she was struck by the fact that there were few moans and groans and hardly any crying. 'They all had big grins across their faces. It's hard to believe but they looked pleased. They were just getting on with fighting their terrible illnesses. Just taking it for granted. They weren't my children, but I felt proud of them all.'

Her daughter was the healthiest-looking child there. Carol was ashamed she'd ever felt sorry for herself and for Alice. All she had to show were a few bruises, but these plucky children seemed very ill indeed. 'I suppose I was beginning to learn what sort of family we'd been until now, selfishly unaware of other people's problems.'

This time, seeing children of her own age undergoing treatment did not perturb Alice. She eagerly joined other youngsters at the play table, helping them to make a tall tower from brightly coloured plastic bricks. Later, when 'Dr Mike' called their name, Alice pushed up eagerly from the table. But the doctor told her, 'It's all right, Alice, you carry on playing. It's just your mum and dad I want to see this time.'

'Dean and I glanced at each other. We knew we were about to be told bad news; otherwise why would Alice be excluded? My heart fluttered, missed a beat.' A wary expression also crept into Alice's face. Perhaps she expected her parents to disappear through the door into 'Dr Mike''s office, never to return. 'You'll come back and get me, won't you, Mum?' she called out, plaintively. Carol imagined her daughter as 'a very small rabbit, with big, brown, frightened eyes'. Play therapist Carol Simpson, who was to become a valuable support to Alice, noticed her distress too. She hurried over to distract her, gently leading her back to the play table.

Outside in the corridor, 'Dr Mike' greeted the couple with a smile. Both noticed it was a sad smile and their hearts fell even more. There was something about the doctor's body language, awkward, stiff and slightly defensive, which alerted them. Once again, Carol wanted to leave everything to Dean. She would rather he spoke to 'Dr Mike' alone, to spare her from hearing grim tidings at first hand. She also had to push aside the now familiar impulse to rush back through the clinic doors, grab Alice and hug her closely. Oppressed by grim foreboding, the couple made their feet follow the doctor through a pair of double doors into another corridor with more doors off it. They trudged along into a small windowless room. It was furnished only with three cheap armchairs and a shabby round coffee table. Even so, Dean thought the chairs seemed too comfortable for painful news.

'Dr Mike' left them alone while he fetched the hospital notes on Alice. Though he seemed a long time, the couple couldn't speak to each other as they waited. But the quiet didn't help. Both were feeling sick. Dean had a premonition that Alice's illness, whatever it was, would be rare and hard to treat, while Carol felt she was somehow outside this horrendous tableau altogether. Her mind left her body and was gazing down from the ceiling at another man and woman she didn't know. She'd had the same peculiar experience when doing exams at school. Then she noticed a solitary print on the wall. She concentrated her gaze on it – a landscape by Monet of a woman and child walking through a field of poppies. Carol drew a small degree of comfort from this sunny scene. Time passed. Then 'Dr Mike' returned, gripping the fateful notes. What awful words did they contain? Dean noticed that the young doctor had opened his mouth and was speaking very slowly. Another bad sign?

'At long last,' he said mildly ' I have a diagnosis for Alice.' They braced themselves. This was it! '*I have a diagnosis for Alice.*' Carol's heart was pounding, her legs literally shaking. Dean felt his hands and feet grow cold. Should they stand up now or take it sitting down? He thought it might be safer to sit. '*I have a diagnosis for Alice.*' They dimly heard the words 'severe aplastic anaemia'. What did he say? What was that? It sounded rather comic.

The doctor repeated himself at Dean's request and this time they both caught the words, 'aplastic anaemia'. They'd heard the illness mentioned before by Dr Chapple in Dewsbury District Hospital. But now it was confirmed by one of the North's foremost children's doctors. From hereon these two words would never be far away from the Maddocks family. Yet at that moment, the name of Alice's illness didn't fill the couple with dread. They still weren't sure what 'aplastic' meant. But they knew anaemia was a shortage of blood and surely that could be treated. Carol had an urge to enfold Alice in her arms and run with her, laughing as she went, through the hospital gates.

However, 'Dr Mike' was still speaking. They both wished the interview would end. They had heard enough for one day. Perhaps he could give them 'part two' tomorrow. Yet they forced themselves to concentrate. 'Alice needs a transplant of bone marrow,' the doctor was saying. 'That's all right then,' thought Dean with a sigh, 'the rest of the family has loads of bone marrow to give her.' But then 'Dr Mike' spoke the worst words of their life: *'If we can't find a match, Alice will have a relatively short life.'*

Instinctively, Dean was defensive. 'I sat there quietly but I was telling myself the man's talking rubbish! How can Alice's life be in danger when she's so fit and full of fun, playing a few yards away just outside your door?' Everything went quiet. The doctor appeared to expect a question. But neither Dean nor Carol could oblige. They didn't want any more evil tidings like that. The doctor was talking again, but perhaps he'd lapsed into a foreign language, because none of it was going in. *'If we can't find a match, Alice will have a relatively short life.'*

Carol had been sitting as still as a statue, almost unable to move let alone speak. 'I was dumb struck. I couldn't have spoken. I couldn't open my mouth to say anything. I was like that for what seemed an age but was probably only several minutes.' As time slowly passed in the small windowless room, Carol began coming out of shock but refused to accept what she'd just heard. When the sympathetic doctor stopped speaking, she firmly but simply replied, 'No, Alice will not have a short life because I will do everything in my power to prevent that. She will not only see her eighth birthday, but she will reach 80 as well!'

When Carol looks back on that bleak day, she recalls, 'I felt like I was being given the most important task a parent could ever receive – to fight for my child's life. And Dean and I would do this for the love of Alice.

'But to do it, I knew we had to be strong and determined. She was a little girl and I wanted our strength and determination to pass on to her. I knew we faced a lifelong fight but I wanted Alice to be positive so it did not affect her mental health. I was swamped by this overwhelming feeling of responsibility that we had to be so careful how we dealt with this, as it could have far-reaching consequences on Alice's personality and how she is able to deal with her fight for her life.'

Carol turned to 'Dr Mike' and made the simple but heartrending plea, 'Tell us how to save Alice and we will do everything possible. But she won't die.'

* * *

The doctor wasn't taken aback. Parents reacted in different ways to the kind of devastating news he was used to giving. Some wept; some were too pole-axed to say anything; occasionally, they seemed resigned in an instant. And quite a few, like Carol, refused to accept his news and became defiant. He did all he could ever do at such times: he said he was sorry. Such interviews were the worst part of being a children's doctor. He hated them. And he felt so very sorry for all the parents.

The Maddocks had nothing more to add. They were too disturbed to think of questions. These could wait. Carol wanted to look at fields and wild flowers and sky, to fasten her eyes on something that was nothing to do with doctors and nurses and blood tests and platelets and hospitals. But only pale blue walls faced her, no windows. She couldn't breathe. She couldn't even look at Dean.

When we receive news so dire that it threatens our very life or that of a loved one, we seek protection in high optimism. We refuse to allow our thoughts to progress through to the final awful conclusion. We simply can't countenance an event that would take away our child, together with all our family happiness. Instead, ways of avoiding the catastrophe crowd our consciousness. We clutch at lifelines along the way, just as we would if we fell down an abyss with outcropping vegetation on its walls. We feel, and expect, that any one of those green tufts, if grabbed quickly enough, will save us from the grisly results of our fatal fall. There had to be green tufts the couple could grab to return the family to happy normality.

Carol and Dean stood stock-still to listen intently to how 'Dr Mike' proposed to treat Alice. But they heard none of those plans, because their minds somehow barred their entry. His earlier warning that Alice might have a short life was discarded altogether; it was simply not a possibility. Parents were buried by their children, it was unthinkable it could be the other way round. It would NOT be the other way round. Not for Alice.

The couple returned through the double doors to the playroom wearing insincere grins. Alice saw through their expressions. She immediately asked, 'Well, what did he say?' Her parents lied. 'He says you'll have to take a bit of medicine, but everything will be OK.' They felt awful about that, but could think of nothing else to say.

Severe Aplastic Anaemia

Though they'd acted impulsively by telling 'Dr Mike' they would fight to preserve Alice's life, Dean and Carol soon began doing exactly that. In a few short months, this struggle was to grow to epic proportions and reap fabulous results, turning the family into a modern legend. But their campaign to keep Alice alive and well at all costs began with the tiny step of logging onto the Internet. Search engines pointed to helpful medical websites, which in turn provided reams of notes on severe aplastic anaemia. They sat up in bed night after night, digesting pages of unnerving detail. They read bits out to each other. 'But though we studied it, and eventually understood all the nasty details, we still couldn't believe this rare condition had anything to do with Alice,' said Dean.

They learned that severe aplastic anaemia affects only two in a million children. Adults can develop the symptoms, too, mainly the over-sixties, but the effects are more serious in children.

Though it comes as a surprise to many people, blood is chiefly made by cells in our marrow, the stuff inside our bones. Severe aplastic anaemia stops the bone marrow doing its job of manufacturing two different types of blood content – red cells and white cells. It also stops the production of platelets, essential agents that help the blood to clot.

As it can no longer produce components of blood, the bone marrow ends up with far too many fat cells. This condition is known as aplasia, which is where the 'aplastic' bit comes in. But why does the bone marrow stop producing blood cells in the first place? The startling answer is that it comes under attack from the patient's own immune system. It's not known why this happens, except that agents known as lymphocytes which are supposed to see off germs, somehow become confused as to what they're supposed to be doing.

To bring the blood back to normal levels, the patient needs donations of both red blood cells and platelets. This can't continue forever though, because transfusions can build up harmful levels of iron in the body. Aplastic anaemia sufferers can be treated with drugs that suppress the body's immune system. Then it no longer has the power to attack the bone marrow. The trouble is that once his or her natural protection is weakened, the patient is vulnerable to all sorts of serious infections. This makes the alternative – a donation of bone marrow – so important to Alice. It could soon return her to health.

Blood-making cells that have been damaged or destroyed by the immune system can't be replaced by the patient's own body. But a donation of exactly the right match of bone marrow would replace these cells and provide a cure. Unfortunately, with Alice the chances of finding a donor are not high because her marrow is an especially rare type. And that's why building up the British bone marrow registers was to become such an urgent undertaking for Carol and Dean. The more volunteers on the books, the greater the chance of finding the right donor to save their daughter.

One of the most distressing facts the couple learned about severe aplastic anaemia is that it shares the same symptom as haemophilia, the well-known inherited condition, which stops the blood clotting. This means that the smallest cut can lead to a dangerous loss of blood. An internal injury will also cause serious problems, as blood fails to congeal inside the body. Such bleeding can easily go unnoticed – until severe damage has been done. There's another danger too. A small bump on the head could cause a an unstoppable haemorrhage that might either kill Alice or cause brain damage.

The effect of this devastating symptom on the Maddocks family can easily be imagined. 'We knew we would be living in fear from now on,' said Carol. 'Something as ordinary as a nosebleed is unstoppable. The slightest scratch is serious. We need to be alert every minute of each day. And how dare we leave Alice with anyone else, even for a moment? We try not to think about it, but it's hard. Alice lives in a cocoon. It's a horrible position to be in.'

After boning up on severe aplastic anaemia, the couple were in mental turmoil. It was hard not to think of Alice's illness every minute of the day. Yet, though they'd been plunged into an abyss of depression and worry, they knew ordinary life had to carry on as usual. Going to work, taking the sisters to and from school, doing the washing, cleaning the house. Everything had to continue normally, or Alice would forfeit the raptures of childhood in a joyless exchange for a life of incessant worry.

The Strawberry Incident

This conflict between coping with the dire news of Alice's illness and the usual domestic routine had some odd effects. It showed, for instance, in the first trip the family made to Sainsbury's after hearing the final diagnosis. Carol was usually very careful to check prices, but now she was on automatic pilot, piling up items in her trolley without proper thought. Her creaking trolley was already in danger of overload, when she distractedly picked up a punnet of strawberries. Dean didn't approve. He tutted and murmured, 'Do we really need these strawberries?' Carol thought this behaviour very odd. She was constantly thinking deeply about Alice's future and wasn't in a mood to tolerate an argument over a few silly strawberries. She would rather Dean kept the girls under tighter control as, without their mother's usual discipline, they were noisily careering around the aisles.

When the checkout bill totalled more than £150, Dean went on the boil. He began ranting, 'All that money on food! It's ridiculous! For one thing, we don't need those bloody strawberries.' Carol found this scene at the front of a long queue very embarrassing. She seethed with anger, but didn't say anything as Dean continued to simmer on the way back to the car. He carefully counted each strawberry as Carol struggled to pack the boot. 'Do you realise,' he asked Carol as they drove home, 'how much those bloomin' strawberries were?'

'I'm not really interested.'

'Well, they were 35p each!'

'Fancy!'

Back home, the two girls stayed in the car – they were due to go on to their granny's for tea – while Carol and Dean relayed carrier bags into the kitchen. He was still bridling about the price of strawberries. Carol snapped, 'I picked up the punnet and hurled it straight at Dean.' An ominous whirring sound split the air. Dean moved too late. Soft ripe fruit slid down his face, his neat cotton shirt and his trousers. Shocked, he jumped aside, leaving a human outline in juicy pink on the kitchen wall. He looked like he'd gone face down into a tray of jam. 'There,' she cried in glee, 'they're not worth bloody anything now, are they?'

This released enough tension to start a feisty row, Carol screaming that Dean should be more concerned about Alice than a few strawberries. Dean, on the other hand, fiercely opined that Carol should be more careful on how they spend their money in future. The upshot of this vigorous up-and-downer was that an angry Dean drove the children to his mother's, leaving Carol pacing up and down the kitchen. But now on her own, with the chance to think things through clearly, Carol realised that investing importance in such a triviality was Dean's way of pushing Alice's illness onto the backburner. 'I knew he'd never normally be bothered about the cost of a few strawberries. Dean is a generous man. Nor would I have thrown them at him. It was the first and last time such a thing has happened but it showed the strain we were under. It's probably why so many couples split up under similar pressures. Fortunately for us, and more importantly for Chloe and Alice, our marriage is as strong as a tank,' says Carol. 'and we've had strawberries many times since – and always served with a smile.'

* * *

As if one wasn't enough, two more domestic dramas were to strike the family that night. Both in their different ways were very unpleasant...

A few hours after their row, now reconciled but tired, the couple smelt something very disagreeable in their house. They wandered into their living room to discover the source of the hideous stench. Their new carpet, a rare expensive purchase, was newly covered in scattered and smelly piles of pooh and vomit. The culprit wasn't far away. Alice's beloved white West Highland terrier Mac had suddenly forgotten he was house-trained. He looked at them with despairing eyes.

Carol guessed that the little dog had had a stroke. She wanted to ring for immediate help. But Dean's recently discovered parsimony surfaced again. He refused to call a vet at night, because of the extra expense. A second row erupted, something on the lines of 'you never liked dogs, anyway'. This time Dean stood his ground, and after making Mac comfortable (he didn't seem in pain), they held their noses, scrubbed away at the appalling mess and tried not to be sick. They didn't know it yet, but the night's trouble had only just begun...

No sooner had they crawled exhausted into bed than Dean started rubbing his chest. 'I think I've got a bit of indigestion.'

'Are you sure it's indigestion?'

'Well, I think it is.'

'Are you sure, though?'

'How do I know?'

The discomfort grew. Dean started to rub his arm. Sharp pain invaded his shoulder and then moved to a new home at the top of his spine. Carol was alarmed. 'That's it, get up, get up. What if you're having a heart attack? You'll have to go to hospital.'

'I'm not going to hospital. I've had enough of them,' Dean snapped.

'Well, I'm not waking up next to a corpse in the morning! So get up.'

'I won't.'

'Up...now!'

A call was made to Dean's mother to come and look after the two girls, while the couple sped off in wind and horizontal rain to Dewbury District Hospital. They braced themselves for a late Friday night in the infamous accident and emergency department. But even Dean, no stranger to the world of drunks and drug addicts, was aghast at the disorderly scenes before them. The place was full of ruffians. Unkempt patients were staggering about, demanding attention, screaming. Obscenities were hurled at doctors and nurses. One man had grabbed a medic by his white coat, threatening to go home for a knife to 'do him in'. There were frenetic attempts to save a pregnant woman who had taken an overdose.

'It was like one of those medieval paintings of Hell, absolutely horrendous,' Carol recalls. 'And this is what the staff in these places have to put up with most nights. I was so sorry for them; they were tremendous.' But the drunk and disorderly scenes around them weren't the only things to worry about.

When Dean explained his symptoms, a duty doctor took the view that Carol's guess was right – he could indeed be having a heart attack. Resuscitation equipment was sent for. He was hurriedly connected to an electrocardiogram machine to check the beat. By now Carol felt she was the heroine of a horror film that was out of control. She'd recently been told her daughter's life was threatened by a rare illness nobody had heard of. The dog had done foul things to her home. And now it seemed her husband would perish at any moment.

Carol stayed with a deeply worried Dean until 4 a.m.; he was then transfered to a ward and Carol went home. Dean was ordered to stay in hospital. His heart was still 'a matter of concern' to the doctors. That didn't help him to sleep.

* * *

In the morning, Carol took poor Mac to the vet's. Sadly, her instincts were proved right again. Alice's little pet had had a stroke and Carol, with a heavy heart, agreed he should be put down. As she drove home, she was beginning to think that for the Maddocks, news of the worst kind was now emerging from every corner – a view confirmed when she walked through the front door. She was greeted by Dean's mother Joan, who, after staying overnight with the girls, had remained to do the housework. 'I'm sorry,' she began inauspiciously. 'I don't know how to begin, but I've got something really awful to tell you...'

Carol felt icy fingers tickle their way up her spine and back again. 'I thought Dean had died and was speechless. But his mother had a different kind of bad news to give me.'

Joan hesitantly explained, 'I was vacuuming the kitchen floor and somehow a large corner of its vinyl covering vanished up the nozzle. I'm really sorry, Carol.'

The older woman was alarmed to see her daughter-in-law sink to her knees, both hands clasping her slowly nodding head. She seemed to be having a breakdown. But it was only relief. She hauled herself to her feet, and then escaped to her bedroom to make up a few hours' lost sleep. When she woke, she found that her good-natured, hard-working mother-in-law had ironed all the creases out of Alice's favourite party dress. Sadly, those creases were a feature of the design, making this expensive gift really special. Carol broke into violent sobs. She'd not cried for Alice's diagnosis, the dog's stroke or Dean's heart problem. But the ruined child's dress was the final straw. She cried uncontrollably for some time. Deciding that consolation was pointless, Dean's mother left silently in a bit of a hurry.

* * *

Later, waking to the misty shape of Carol materialising by his hospital bed, Dean was surprised to find himself being told off. 'You're sitting here like Lord Muck,' cried Carol vehemently. 'But what about me! I have to sort out all these problems at home. And it's all your fault in the first place. If you hadn't got yourself into a state about some stupid strawberries, none of this would have happened.'

Dean wished his vocal visitor would leave him. 'I don't need this while I'm in here,' he mumbled under his breath. He was glad the doctors had put him down for at least another night, so he could have some peace. But after 48 hours on the ward, Dean was sent off home with a warning. His heart should stay healthy, they said, as long as he didn't get too stressed. Dean was to look back on this warning with some amusement – the unremitting strain of the next few years would be almost unbearable.

So far as the 'heart attack' went, Dean thought the experts were worrying unduly. He'd never had problems with his health before and he put his pains down to a pulled muscle ... caused by trying to dodge flying strawberries. Carol also takes a sanguine view of that weekend's disasters. 'The main tragedy of our lives, the threat to Alice, was something we believe we coped with quite well, considering the seriousness of it and how alien it all was to us. But it left us no energy to deal with the minor hiccups. Those we made a complete hash of.'

As is often the way with children, the loss of Mac, the West Highland terrier, didn't seem to upset Alice too much. But a week later, her mother found a note in her bedroom. It was addressed to 'Mac in Heaven'.

Dear Mac,
I love you and I will forever. I am missing you a lot. Are you feeling better? I hope you are safe with God. You will be, don't worry.
From your best buddy, Alice.
PS I will be with you soon, so wait up.

Carol felt tears sting her cheeks as she read the words: 'I was cleaning her bedroom when I came across the note. It frightened me. Did Alice really think she might die? Dean and I never admitted the possibility, even to ourselves. I spent the rest of the day in her bedroom, listening to her favourite CDs, looking at her trinkets, absorbing every bit of her. The smell of her pillow, perfumes she used, all her little girlie things. Once I'd cleaned the room, I lay on her bed. I was really mournful, depressed. I wept loads and prayed.

'I thought a lot about my mum. For the first time, I realised what she must have felt for us, what being a mother was about and how I'd taken it for granted. I wondered if my mum had ever worried about me like this, but she wasn't here for me to ask. Alice was a year old when Mum died aged 58 from a brain haemorrhage. It was the third she'd had but her death was still sudden.

'I stayed in Alice's room all day until it was time to pick the girls up. I put on make-up, got ready and anyone who met me that afternoon would not have known a thing was wrong. It did me good to wallow in my own pity. Many times since, I've spent a few hours in Alice's room. It gives me some comfort. It's like she is there but in the stillness and quiet, not in her usual bustling way.'

That afternoon, Carol held onto the note and pondered over their lives. They'd certainly tried hard to keep their daughter from the darkness still to come. Yet here, in a scribbled note to her pet dog, Alice seemed to understand and have some acceptance that she might not have long to live. It was a harrowing moment.

The Big Test

The following week, Dean, Carol and Chloe were due at St. James's Hospital for an important milestone. Tests would be done to see if any of them could be bone marrow donors for Alice. Chloe was the best hope – there was a one-in-four chance of a sister's bone marrow doing the trick. The odds fell to one-in-six for parents. Carol was greatly anxious about asking Chloe to give a sample. It could be tricky. Her elder daughter was frightened of hospitals, even more so since Alice's illness. What if she said no? What then? They would have to make her. They had no choice about that. But it would be awful to force Chloe to take the test. Carol thought for a long time before deciding how to approach the older girl. She kept putting the moment off.

Then, as Chloe was getting undressed for a bath, she asked Carol, 'Is Alice going to get well?'

'Yes, but we have to help her. We have to find somebody with the right bone marrow.'

Carol explained that bone marrow was a liquid inside our bones that helps to make our blood. Alice's bone marrow wasn't doing its job, and had to be changed with some more – from a healthy person. Sometimes a sister was just the right person to give a bit of bone marrow. Would Chloe like to do that?

'Yes,' she said simply and climbed into the bath. 'Thank goodness,' thought Carol contentedly.

But later that evening, Carol found Chloe crying softly in her bed. 'Come on, darling, get into our bed and Dad will get into yours,' said Carol. This was routine when either of the girls were upset during the night. Neither of them slept. Carol reassured her that there was nothing to worry about; that they would all be tested at the same time.

When the family arrived at St James's, poor Chloe was shaking. Alice on the other hand was smug. 'I don't know what the matter with you all. It's dead easy. It's only a little prick.' 'Dr Mike' took Chloe's hand and promised softly, 'I won't hurt you.' Chloe was greatly surprised when he didn't.

Carol was strangely excited immediately after the three samples had been taken. In fact, both parents were in an exuberant mood. They were sure Chloe would have perfectly matching bone marrow, even if they hadn't. After all, allowing for the two and a half years' age difference, the sisters were strikingly alike. They shared similar looks, pastimes and personalities. Surely they would share the same bone marrow.

But it was an odd kind of confidence. Nothing was guaranteed, after all. So much depended on these tests. If just one of the threesome could provide a precise match for Alice, as they all so confidently expected, then a life-giving transfer could be made. But if not, a search would have to be made for an outside donor, an uncertain process that could take years, and may not bear fruit until too late.

* * *

The test results wouldn't be ready for two weeks. To ease the waiting, the family spent a few days at Dean's parents' caravan near Bridlington on the Yorkshire coast. They tried to forget the tests in the weak sunshine, and of course, failed miserably. But they did stay optimistic. On the drive back, Carol was contented for the first time since Alice had fallen over in her friend's garden two months before. Though there was only that one-in-four chance of Chloe supplying a perfect match, she was still certain of success. 'I felt God would answer my prayers,' she said. 'Chloe would be the perfect donor.' She began to hum a pop tune, but not everybody in the car was cheerful. Alice was carsick.

Carol's happy mood was obliterated when they were summoned to St James's to learn from 'Dr Mike' that Chloe's marrow was not the same type as Alice's. Neither was that of either of her parents. There was shocked silence. 'We felt so let down. One part of me was relieved for Chloe because I knew she was so frightened of having an operation. She would have done anything for her sister but it still didn't stop her being scared. But the other part of me felt angry. It was a massive blow to us.'

It was indeed a vicious setback. Alice would now need intensive drug treatment to subdue her immune system and stop it attacking her bone marrow. So complex and hazardous was the regime planned for her, that Alice would need to be carefully monitored during a long spell in hospital. Meanwhile, a world search would begin for a suitable donor. There was still hope – of course there was – but Alice's chances of survival were seriously reduced by the negative result of the tests. Dean and Carol felt a mallet had hit them. They'd been beaten down by one delivery of bad news after another. In the space of a few weeks, they'd been cruelly changed from a carefree, lively family into a very worried, careworn one, cursed with the prospect of dreadful things awaiting them.

When Chloe was told her bone marrow wasn't the same as her sister's, Dean expected her to be relieved. She had escaped the intimidating operation of having bone marrow taken from her back. But Chloe didn't smile. 'She told us she was really disappointed. Being Chloe, she'd wanted to help Alice, whatever it took,' says Dean.

The family now had to prepare themselves for a gruelling regime of hospital treatment for Alice to stop her immune system attacking her bone marrow. Carol and Dean, who'd assumed the relevant drugs were man-made, were strangely disturbed to find they were in fact lymphocytes taken from human blood. These are special fighting cells whose normal job is to neutralise viruses in the body. To be effective in Alice's treatment, they would first be injected into rabbits before being introduced directly into her blood supply. The animals' metabolism conveniently alters the cells to make them more effective when later used to suppress Alice's immune system.

'Dr Mike' warned the couple the treatment might make their daughter very ill. Alice, of course, was not told this or indeed anything else about her treatment, except that once she went to hospital she would be there for 'quite a bit'.

A Girl Like Alice

Alice has never understood just how serious her illness is. As the months go by, Dean and Carol have not told her 'Dr Mike's warning that her life could be short.'

'She doesn't need to know,' says Carol. 'She's just a child and it's our responsibility to keep her thinking positively. She loves school. She loves everything about life. And it upsets her when she sees other sick children in hospital.'

This confident declaration hides some confusion in Carol's mind. The truth is that from the moment aplastic anaemia was identified, neither parent had ever been sure quite how to play it. They decided to represent Alice's disorder as an exciting chance for her to help other children in the same boat. They've also told her that if she cannot find a suitable bone marrow donor for herself, then it doesn't matter: she would still be able to have blood transfusions forever.

Sadly, this is not the case, as frequent blood transfusions lead to a damaging build-up of iron.

Alice is a child with a hungry mind. She compels her parents to find more answers than they want to give. Consequently, they find it more and more difficult to filter out alarming facts, without resorting to lies that could backfire in the future. To help Alice understand how important it is to keep looking for a donor, Carol told her, 'These blood transfusions are a bit of a nuisance, Alice. But if we can get you a bone marrow transplant, it means you can travel to lovely places when you grow up.' She warmed to the theme. 'You can also do more sport. At the moment you can't because you get bruises and you bleed easily.'

At first Dean and Carol didn't realise how difficult it would be to find exactly the right match. As this fact slowly dawned on them, they never explained to Alice just how dangerous the situation really was. Yet strangely, even when the time comes to tell their daughter just how grave her disorder is, they don't expect her to be frightened or distressed. 'Amazingly, she's just accepted things the way they are,' said Carol proudly. 'To Alice, her illness is one of those things. And no matter how bad the news we give her, it will just be water off a duck's back.'

* * *

Alice is grateful to her parents for their unending struggle to find a donor. For example, she entered a competition in a comic inviting children to nominate their mum to be a 'queen for a day'. With considerable help from Chloe, Alice wrote, 'Our mum is a lady who many people have noticed for her way of standing up for something that she deeply believes in. She is the flower that stands out from the bunch. If the sun doesn't shine or she hasn't been watered, she'll carry on till she gets there. She is the blossom in the family tree. She treats us like princesses, so why shouldn't she be a queen?'

But stoical and caring though Alice is, she can be obstinate. 'She sometimes revels in being downright awkward,' says Carol. 'In fact, she can be a right little madam!' In the thick of one of the family's darker periods, Carol remembers a big rumpus over what Alice should wear to a christening service. Carol had a smart party dress in mind, but Alice wanted to go in jeans and T-shirt. There were sobs, answerings-back and heavy stamping of feet before Carol finally had her way. There are many stormy scenes like that. 'In one way it's quite nice, because it's so normal to have mother and daughter arguments,' she said.

But at the same time Carol always feels some remorse. 'How can I rave at Alice when she's so desperately ill? What if she died tomorrow? I'd have to remember all my life how I'd just shouted at her and made her cry. How could I stand that?'

Both Carol and Dean understand they have to be firm with their vulnerable, breakable daughter. Otherwise, illness or no illness, she could turn into a selfish, demanding child. They know it's doubly important not to give into Alice because other people naturally try to be nice to her. They give her presents and organise treats in a misplaced attempt to compensate for her affliction. Some of these kind folk are celebrities. Alice finds herself the centre of attention in glamorous places, like radio stations and television studios. To turn her into a classic spoilt brat would be inevitable if her parents weren't strict. 'If we'd never told her off or pulled her into line, we'd have a "Child from Hell" on our hands by now,' Dean explained.

* * *

Keeping her on a tight rein has turned Alice into a well-balanced, self-reliant child. She is also, when her precarious health allows, full of energy. In between hospital treatments and their draining after-effects, Alice tries to make up for lost time. 'She always gets the most out of the few occasions she feels well,' said Dean. 'She likes to paint or make things with sticky tape, coloured tissue paper and all that. But she's never demanding of us, just happy to get on with things by herself.' She has an impish sense of humour too, not above leaving secret Mickey Mouse impressions on the answering machine.

These days, Alice's very dark brown eyes normally show signs of tiredness. But just mention the word 'school' and a brilliant smile brightens her pale face. The most annoying thing for Alice about her illness is that her many hospital visits get in the way of lessons. Mum and Dad often have to ignore the doctor's advice and allow her to whizz back to school after treatment, when she should really be resting at home. It's as though she's anchored to her desk by invisible elastic. When other children are ill, the staff phone their parents to suggest they're taken home. But teachers are reluctant to do that with Alice. They've learnt that if they do call Carol or Dean, Alice just refuses to go. She usually climbs into her blue check dress about an hour before she needs to walk to school in the morning. Her favourite lessons are art and maths. But what she really enjoys is interacting with her friends.

There are 130 pupils in Hanging Heaton's junior and infants school. Their head teacher, Bev Drury proudly affirms that, given Alice's condition, she couldn't be in a better place. 'Everyone here, staff and children alike, regards Alice as someone special.' She describes her pupil as kind, modest, hard-working and full of perseverance. But her most striking quality is her cheerful energy. 'You wouldn't believe it, considering all she's been through, but she always forcing herself on. She's a diligent, delightful child. And we feel privileged that she's here.' Though her illness has robbed her of many lessons, Alice, attentive and quick on the uptake, still manages to beat the average in most subjects. Her last report showed nine As and two Bs.

Teachers and pupils take care not to mention her illness. Carol has asked the staff to treat Alice exactly as an ordinary little girl. They discreetly passed this request to her classmates – and now Alice has no sense of receiving any special treatment. Yet the staff are on alert. If she looks tired, they suggest she sits down in their common room. They're quick to step in if a rough game develops, so Alice doesn't get a chance to cut herself. The teachers know the blood would be hard to stop. For two years, Alice wasn't allowed to do PE, but she was so disappointed, she's now allowed to join in. Secretly the gym teacher makes sure she's not put in harm's way.

Alice even insisted that she took part on sports day. The longest race of the afternoon was around the large school field. Dean and Carol sat at the side of the sports field. 'We watched all the children take part in the run. When Alice insisted she also took part, Dean and I decided to run along behind her just to keep an eye on her. We felt so proud of her determination and strength to keep going but we were also hoping she was going to be OK. Puffing gamely and not keeping a very straight line, Alice began to run out of steam, but was determined to finish. Forty yards behind everyone else, she ended the race to tremendous applause. Dean and I both had tears in our eyes as she proudly yelled to us all, "I did it. I did it!"'

Teachers have been amazed that Alice's disorder hasn't affected her personality one jot. 'She was a delightful child before – and she still is now,' said her head teacher, Bev Drury. 'All the attention lavished on her by the media, all the famous people she's met has no effect whatever. She's modest, doesn't boast about anything, never shows off.'

Alice also seems unperturbed by her illness, the nastiness of her treatment and the fact that she's frequently and without warning whisked into hospital for more blood transfusions. 'She's stoical and she accepts it,' said Mrs Drury. 'Nobody, and I mean nobody, hears her complain.'

Chloe

If Alice is sensitive to the needs of those around here, Chloe can take the credit for showing her how. Alice couldn't have a better sister to help her cope with her illness. She's one of those rare children: a carer and sharer. Assistants noticed this happy trait in the nursery. If a toddler fell or bumped into something, Chloe would run across the room with a hankie to wipe away the tears. She took other little mites to the toilet, or brought them cups of orange squash. She amused the staff by buttoning up children's coats at going home time. She is Alice's best friend, and they have spent hours playing together, often in the battered and much-loved Wendy house at the bottom of the garden. Chloe is well suited to her role as a constant hospital visitor. She's patient and tolerant. Nobody has a bad word for Chloe Maddocks.

My Sister Alice

You are my unique sister
A really special soul,
And in my life you've always
Played a very special role.

I wonder if you really know
Just how loved you are,
Because for all who know you
You're a bright and shining star.

I feel so lucky you're my sister
And I really hope you know,
You'll always mean the world to me
Wherever I may go.

The future is something
That we have yet to explore,
But with the two of us I'm sure
There'll be some fun in store.

Love, Clo Jo

Though she's now left Alice's village school to go to the local comprehensive, Bev Drury will never forget Chloe's ability to put her own needs last. 'It's an astounding trait,' she says. 'I've never seen the like.'

The caring qualities of Chloe have developed with age. At her first 'parent's evening' at Woodkirk High School, her science teacher, went over to Dean and Carol with a stunning endorsement of their older child's character. 'I wanted to tell you what a lovely child you have. Academically, she's a star. But as a young person, she's a superstar. She's loving and kind, never belittles anybody and is always willing to help her classmates, who may not be as capable as her.'

Dean and Carol swelled with pride. Science teachers in comprehensives aren't known for their generosity of praise. For one of the critical breed to seek them out during a busy open evening to say such fine things about Chloe, meant a lot. All parents think their children special, but here was independent evidence of the first order.

When Chloe visits Alice in hospital, she's always on the look out for children whose parents aren't there. Then she sits with them, helps to colour a picture or – as she used to do in the nursery – brings them some orange squash.

If Chloe hadn't been blessed with a generous heart, it would have been very difficult for her parents. Because Alice needs so much hospital treatment, they're often forced to leave Chloe with relatives and friends. Most children react to that by being naughty to attract more attention. Occasionally Chloe does that – but very rarely and never for long.

Emergencies on Ward 10

The schools broke up; house martins swooped along the streets in Hanging Heaton; middle-aged men put on shorts and looked ridiculous; and Alice's long summer stay in Ward 10, the children's cancer ward at St James's Hospital, was about to begin. The ward is situated in the Gledhow Wing, a modern six-storey building, with a florist, a bank, a W.H. Smith and a big clattery cafeteria. Lifts take you to the fourth floor where Ward 10 is the temporary home for young cancer patients and children like Alice who have serious blood disorders.

Dean pushed an intercom button to announce their arrival. Suspicious eyes inspected him on the video camera before the family was admitted. The door clicked behind them, Carol remembers, 'like the door of a condemned cell'. Once inside, the atmosphere lightened; they heard the chatter of children and they felt better. The walls were a cheerful sky blue. Off the main corridor were a number of open plan areas, known as 'bays', each containing four children's beds. Every bay was painted in a different colour, the yellow and green ones more welcoming than the angrier red and the colder blue.

Dean and Carol were shocked to see an enormous notice board, covered with about fifty photos of young patients. Each child had a note of their illness, and the date of their diagnosis. There were 'thank-you' letters to staff on the board, too. And newspaper clippings telling of fund-raising events held by well-wishers to send the children on holiday. Though the board was clearly meant to encourage, it did the opposite for Dean and Carol. It brought home to them the large number of local children who were perilously ill.

With staged gaiety, Dean and Carol brought Alice into the ward with her pyjamas and toothbrush, while Chloe trotted behind to keep her company. Chloe was edgy. Trying to hide behind her father, she was wondering unhappily if her sister would soon lose her shiny dark brown hair, like most of the children playing around them. But Alice took the older girl's hand and said, 'Come on, Chloe. There's nothing to be scared of.' She led her big sister to a table where young patients were colouring pictures. Chloe noticed that most of them were 'very pale and poorly'. A bed was found for Alice, her soft toys were arranged at the end of it, and Dean and Carol prepared to spend their nights in a fold-away bed beside her.

The treatment itself had an unhappy start. It began with a blood transfusion. It was only one of hundreds Alice was to need, but it was the most harrowing. She was taken from the ward to a day clinic some distance away for the transfusion to take place. But it was ill-timed. Though the transfusion, a much slower procedure than most of us realise, needed to continue until the early evening, the clinic was closed as usual at 5 p.m. So a small procession then wound its way from the clinic through the complex corridors and grounds of one of the Britain's biggest hospitals back to the distant Ward 10. A nurse in a spotless uniform, bustling and efficient, propelled Alice in a wheelchair. Alongside, Carol pushed a metal stand on wheels with the blood transfusion gear on it. Linking the two contraptions was a wobbly tube anchored in Alice's arm. Both women had to walk at exactly the same speed.

The distance between the two hospital sites is about a quarter of a mile. At one point, this odd vision had to cross a busy road and go down a weed-strewn, uneven path. The summer sun scorched down. As usual at St James's, there were hundreds of people about. Carol remembered, 'Alice didn't like it. She didn't want people looking at her. And we felt uncomfortable because they were all staring. We passed through one area, a rehabilitation unit of some sort, where a gang of drug addicts or drunks were being rowdy and unpleasant.' There was nothing Carol could do to shield Alice from this unwholesome sight. 'They were pointing to us and smirking. Alice squirmed with embarrassment and shame. It was a horrible thing for a child who'd never even been in a wheelchair before.'

At last, they took the final lift to Ward 10. 'Dr Mike' had earlier warned Carol that some children on the ward were now in the later stages of their lives and that Alice might be distressed to see them. Carol watched her daughter anxiously. Alice was miles away, lost in thought. Suddenly, she turned to her mother, 'You won't let them take my hair, will you? Please can we go home?'

Carol nearly cracked then. She longed to pull out the drip and end this torture. 'I thought to hell with it. We're not putting her through this any more. We're going home.' Instead she put her arm round Alice and said mildly, 'Doctors don't take the hair, love. It's the medicine that takes the hair. The children without hair are getting better, because they're having the right medicine to make them well.'

Alice began to cry softly. Her long hair was her pride. She loved more than anything to comb and plait it. She and Chloe would sit for hours playing hair stylists. How, she wondered, could she play at hairdressers without any hair?

* * *

The sight of Alice in tears plunged Carol into her blackest despair since the family's ordeal began ten weeks earlier. She was beginning to realise for the first time that this malevolent illness could be fatal. 'I was in a deep depression, wondering why. Why Alice? Why us? I felt that all four of us were going to slaughter in an unknown world. I was full of terror. I wasn't safe.'

She drifted quietly away from Alice, who was now playing happily with hospital toys. For a while she sat alone in a corner of a playroom, part of Ward 10. 'I huddled on this tiny kiddie's chair and felt like a child again, helpless against a hideous and desolate future.' Then she succumbed to even darker fears, a cold, empty, overpowering feeling of doom. 'This huge responsibility, landed on us from nowhere, was just too heavy to bear. We couldn't possibly cope – and Alice would probably die.'

She sat still for a few minutes, too unhappy and tired to move. Abruptly, and with a bang, the door crashed open and a little boy of about five tore into the playroom. He wore white pyjamas with grey elephants on. He dragged two drip-stands along with him. Each stand had more than one bag on it, each containing a medical fluid of some sort. Some were clear, some coloured. He also had a thickish rubber tube protruding from his stomach. Various electrical wires were attached to other parts of his slight body. Carol saw that he had a grey cardboard bowl under one arm. She'd seen children carry these around the hospital, in case the drugs made them sick.

The tiny patient made his way to a far corner. Still with his bowl under his arm, and hindered by the two laden drip-stands, he dragged a chair bigger than himself towards a rack of tall shelves crammed with toys. He tried scrambling onto a table to reach the top shelf.

Carol, jerking out of her misery, yelled, 'Stop what are you doing! Come down, You're going to hurt yourself!' The boy pointed towards a colourful box and weakly told her, 'I want that up there.' It was a game called Tumblin' Monkeys. Carol reached up to the top shelf and gave the box to the little chap. And, as she did so, she felt ashamed.

'How could I sit there, feeling so sorry for myself,' she reflected afterwards, 'when this little soldier, struck down by what was obviously a very serious illness, was quite happy living with it? And I mean "living". He was determined, wasn't he? Determined to get on with it. He wasn't going to let poor health take away his childhood. Wonderful! That little boy will never know it, but he was my inspiration.'

This incident, more than all the other dramatic events still to come, helped Carol to build both physical and emotional strengths to face the future – and fight it. Her encounter with a five-year-old cancer patient also convinced Carol that she was not somehow being punished by Alice's condition. If this young innocent, now so happily engrossed in his game, could be afflicted by cancer, how could it possibly be his fault? The little boy's mother, breathless and flustered, rushed into the playroom. Thankful to find her escaped son, she told Carol that he'd been extremely ill the day before and was now on stronger drugs, which seemed to have excited him and made him rebellious.

'She looked knackered,' Carol recalled, 'exhausted and drained. But she was fighting hard for her son. And perhaps for the first time, I realised we were not alone; that many parents were struggling through the same battles and, more likely than not, were doing a better job than we were.'

From then on, Carol would stop being dismayed and discouraged by Alice's illness. Instead, with Dean's constant support, she would battle relentlessly for her survival whatever the cost to their careers, their health and their pockets.

* * *

After Alice's first few days on Ward 10 it was realised that all her many blood transfusions had put a strain on the veins of her arm.

They'd started to shrink under the punishment. To ease this problem, Alice was supplied with a Port-A-Cath. This device is fitted, under a general anaesthetic, to the chest wall under the skin. From it runs a tube, which is connected to a main artery into the heart. Once in place, the device allows blood transfusions or drugs to be introduced directly into Alice's body, without the need for needles in her arms.

Recovering from the short operation to fit the Port-A-Cath, Alice didn't feel at all well. She had a rising temperature, a fluey feeling and pains in her chest. Carol was alarmed, but she was given pain-killers and drugs to reduce the fever. That night Dean stayed with his daughter on the ward. Her high temperature persisted, and another tube was fed into Alice's arm to receive an infusion of antibiotics. This lasted for five days and delayed Alice's treatment a further week. Given the alarming nature of these goings-on for a seven-year-old, Alice amazed her nurses by not complaining once.

Finally, it was time for Alice to receive the immunosuppressive drugs that 'could' put the illness into remission. Firstly, Alice was given a small amount of the drug as a test. It was administered in a saline solution by a drip into the newly fitted Port-A-Cath. While this took place, her parents were disconcerted to see a sinister array of syringes and drugs at the bottom of the bed. These, they were told, were to be brought into use should the treatment cause a heart attack, or a shock so serious to the system that it would effectively shut her body down. The test would take an hour, so Dean and Carol knew that anxiety and fear would grip them for that agonising length of time.

'We were on tenterhooks the whole time,' Carol recalls. 'We tried to make small talk with the doctors and nurses. We chatted about the weather, asked if they'd had a nice weekend, that sort of thing. But the strain was awful. Alice was sitting up nonchalantly in the bed, not feeling anything. Yet a potent drug was being pumped into her slight body, a drug that we knew could kill her.'

Dean found himself considering the old question: should they really be putting Alice through this at all? 'This was a game of Russian roulette with our daughter's life at stake. At any moment something awful might happen. And we knew this wasn't just an exaggerated morbid thought. It was a rock solid fact.'

Mercifully, Alice was unaware of the danger she was in. As she sat up in bed calmly colouring a picture, Carol's eye kept straying to the nearest syringe, spotless and ominous on a tray. It contained adrenaline, filled in advance and ready to plunge into Alice's arm if things went wrong. With ten minutes still to go, the treatment suddenly took a turn for the worse. Alice began to have side effects. She became tired and lethargic. Her face was waxy and translucent. She complained of feeling sick. Her legs, arms and neck began to ache. She was lying on the bed now, suffering. She was given codeine for the pain and an anti-allergy drug. What would happen now? Dean and Carol watched fearfully. But finally, the dreadful hour was up and couple felt they'd got away lightly. Relief broke over them. But of course this was only the beginning. The proper anti-immune treatment was yet to start . . .

* * *

The first two weeks dragged by, as the drugs Alice was taking made her feel lethargic and sick. She had a raging temperature and constant diarrhoea. These side effects were expected and acceptable to the doctors, as long as they didn't get worse. Alice was closely monitored, all sorts of tests being made on her progress. Even her urine was carefully checked. When she went to the toilet, she had to use a bedpan. Much to her indignation, 'Alice M' was pencilled on each cardboard container. 'Why does my name have to be written on it?' she asked Dean. 'Nobody's going to steal it.'

There's a new building called Eckersley House in the hospital grounds. Visitors who need to stay long periods can use it for overnight accommodation, washing and so on. Carol wondered whether she dared to leave Alice to go there for a shower. She did, but it was the fastest shower on record. When she returned she was surprised to find Alice was back to her old self, enjoying herself in the playroom. So far, the anti-immune drugs were behaving themselves. The side effects were under control.

But Dean and Carol were still acutely anxious. They had a lot to worry about. It wasn't long before Chloe started to raise concerns.

She's a deep thinker who, like Dean, keeps her feelings hidden. Carol knew her elder daughter was not coping with the situation, but didn't know how best to handle it. Chloe refused to discuss her feelings, but Carol guessed she was upset at seeing her sister in a hospital bed. She'd been looking forward to an afternoon's shopping with Dean's mother. But Carol and Dean hoped she wouldn't go. They said nothing because they sensed that Chloe was torn between wishing to escape from the ward and not wanting to leave Alice behind. She did in fact go on the shopping expedition, but didn't seem happy about it. Plainly, from now on Chloe's needs also had to be considered despite everything else that was going on. She needed lots of TLC too.

Carol also began having selfish and peculiar thoughts, of which she was ashamed. When Alice was going through a bad patch, crying in her misery, her anguished mother wished some other child on the ward could suffer instead. Yet whenever another young patient was in pain, while Alice seemed better, Carol felt guilty her child wasn't the one in distress. She consoled herself with something she once read in her social workers' manual – 'relentless stress causes irrational thinking'.

* * *

The lack of privacy on Ward 10 irritated the couple to distraction. Dean hated to discuss Alice's condition with other parents – or to hear their heart-breaking stories in return. Said Dean, 'It sounds callous, but we didn't want to chat to anyone. We just wanted peace and quiet, so we could tend to Alice. We didn't care about any other child's diagnosis. Looking back, I feel like a monster, but that's the way we felt at the time. It was our way of coping.'

The family began to resent their stay in Ward 10 more and more. Parents often gathered in the ward's kitchen to gossip. Carol found herself giving this confined room a wide berth. Because if she went in, she was invariably button-holed by another parent in search of sympathy and advice. As a social worker whose job is to talk through other people's problems, Carol found herself automatically counselling parents on how to deal with their misery. 'I could see the weight lifting as I discussed things with them. So at first I encouraged them and comforted them in any way I could. And then they'd leave feeling much better.' But Carol came to loathe her new role. 'As I talked with other unhappy parents, their burdens were somehow shifted onto me. I often left that kitchen in an awful state of depression.' Eventually Carol refused to enter the kitchen at all, leaving Dean to act as both cook and waiter.

The Maddocks family has a very close and increasing circle of relatives and friends. There was a regular stream of visitors, bearing toys and sweets for Alice and bottles of wine for her parents. Aunts, uncles, brothers, sisters and cousins all came and the family was very grateful. But there were also times in the busy ward when Carol longed for solitude. She would hide herself in the parents' room to avoid her visitors, and even to get away from Alice and Dean. 'My head was reeling. It was a very busy place. It was like living in Piccadilly Circus. I just wanted to go home.'

Most of all, the couple hated well-meaning inquiries about Alice. 'The other parents constantly asked about aplastic anaemia,' said Dean. 'They'd never come across it before and couldn't fathom what it was. Not surprising, really, because we still weren't sure ourselves.' It was ignorance of the nature of aplastic anaemia that sometimes led other parents on the ward to say thoughtless things, like, 'At least your little girl has still got some hair', as though Alice was somehow more privileged than their child. This was part of a perverse rivalry that stalked the ward.

'On some days, it was like some macabre competition as to who was suffering most,' Carol remembers with distaste. 'It almost came to, "My child has a worse blood count than your child" or "My boy's much more ill than your girl." I was thinking, "I don't care about your child, I have enough to worry about. Go away!"'

Nobody could get away from the smells in Ward 10. Children under intensive treatment to defeat cancer have to put up with bouts of sickness and diarrhoea. But there were other smells, too, and not just the usual antiseptic whiffs of hospitals, but the intangible, pervasive scent of fear. Carol fancied she could hear terror of the unknown in the parents' voices, too. It's unsettling enough when our own lives hang in the balance, but there's more pressing anxiety over our children's health. It was this deeper dread that every parent knows which gives Ward 10 its atmosphere of menace. A cheerful band of nurses, experts in jolly small talk, works tirelessly to dispel the gloom. But it creeps back at every opportunity, mostly at night.

Even with the bedside curtain tightly pulled around, there was no shutting out the ward's harsher realities. Carol could hear what was happening behind other patients' curtains quite clearly. The whispered concerns of parents, and the soft murmur or wild cries of gravely ill children. These were sounds from hell, never to be forgotten. Alice, who could hear all these goings on as well, was keen to protect her own privacy. She hated doctors examining her, insisting that the curtains be drawn around her bed, even if it was just a nurse checking her temperature. And, always aware of other young patients' feelings, she would ask Carol to close their curtains, too.

* * *

Opposite Alice's bed in a hospital cot was a six-month-old baby, called Nisa. She had a brain tumour that made her almost blind. Alice idolised this infant. She spent hours with her hand through the cot bars, stroking the baby's tiny wrist. Though she knew Nisa was very ill, she hadn't been told she was dying. Alice spent hours rattling Nisa's toys, making silly noises to keep her entertained. The child's parents, who had a large family, often had to return home at night. Alice was very worried by this. 'Mum, will you stay awake and look after Nisa, while her mum and dad aren't here?'

So Carol and Dean took it on themselves to look after the baby, as well as Alice. This wasn't a light undertaking. The nature of Nisa's illness and her treatment meant she was sick three or four times a night. When this happened she could be heard choking and spluttering on vomit at the back of her throat. Dean and Carol were on edge all night as they listened for those alarming tell-tale sounds. When they occurred, one of them would leap towards the cot to ease Nisa onto her side. They would also stab a buzzer to bring nurses rushing from their station at the far end of the long ward.

Nisa's parents soon discovered that the kindly parents opposite their baby's cot were watching out and caring for her in the darkness. 'They were so grateful,' said Carol. 'They knew, because we told them so, that when they were compelled to go home at night to look after their other children, Nisa would be safe.'

The Maddocks could see that nurses were thin on the ground in Ward 10. 'They were incredibly busy all the time, totally stretched,' said Dean. 'They deserved better than that, and so did all the children. But we could do nothing to help, we knew resources were strained to the limit.'

* * *

As the treatment wore on, the Maddocks became aware that the doctors treating Alice had fairly limited experience of severe aplastic anaemia. One admitted it had been some time since the hospital had cared for anyone with such a very rare condition; that the treatment regime had now changed and they were no longer fully familiar with the latest procedures. 'This was really scary, and something we didn't want to know,' said Dean. 'When we asked exactly how Alice was to be treated, we were told it was being done "according to protocol". We were never told what this protocol was. But we worried that she wouldn't be treated as an individual, but by some sort of rigid plan set out in a medical textbook. When you know that your daughter's life is at risk, this is hardly encouraging.' At moments like this, Dean fell into black despair.

But then the family discovered the Robert Ogden Centre, a new building in the hospital grounds for the exclusive use of patients with cancer or other life-threatening illnesses. They found it to be a haven from the busy, hectic cheek-by-jowl life that pervades the rest of St James's Hospital. There are sofas and chairs that swallow you up in luxurious comfort. Tiny water fountains play as tranquil music sweeps through tastefully decorated rooms in a swish contemporary style.

When she was well enough to visit this wonderful place, Alice was spirited away by a 'play therapist' who skilfully entertained her in a side ward, while Dean and Carol were themselves pampered by volunteers. These were mainly elderly ladies, supervised by two paid staff, one of whom was a young blonde-haired woman, quietly spoken, with an impressive knowledge of all kinds of cancer. There was also a library of medical books and computers connected to the

Internet. It surprised the couple that there were as many benefits for carers as for the patients. Carol, for example, took full advantage of aromatherapy sessions and massages. All the family would sometimes sneak out of the ward for a short break in this oasis of calm and they came to regard it as the best bit of their lost summer.

The kitchen for Ward 10 had two roomy refrigerators, a pair of microwave ovens and a two-ring hotplate. But cups and plates were rarely to be found. So one day Carol called in at Ikea and donated a set of teatime crockery to the ward. A few days later, most of this collection had vanished into the bags and pockets of visitors. Now the Maddocks knew why the kitchen was so sparsely equipped. Crime was common in this cramped room. The couple labelled any food they left in the refrigerators with a felt-tipped pen. But that didn't stop it disappearing. Dean drew on his police training to try and nab the culprits, but the investigation yielded no results.

The couple were also wary of some visitors to the ward, whom Carol describes as 'unsavoury'. Dean spotted people he'd previously arrested for acts of violence and theft. The staff nurses frequently reported stolen TV sets, video recorders and even toys. 'You couldn't put anything down, unless you watched it very carefully,' said Dean. 'As if we hadn't enough to worry about, without looking out for wretches who stoop to rob desperately ill children.'

Yet Ward 10 had its compensations. Good-humoured doctors and the tireless nursing staff, together with their cheery assistants, were jewels in a rather rusty crown. Thursday night was Alice's highlight every week. That's when a modern saint came trundling down the ward. She was an auxiliary nurse, slim, middle-aged and bespectacled, with greying hair. Busy and full of fun, ever smiling, salt of the earth. The family knew her only as 'Jolly Trolley', though she was more like 'The Pied Piper', as a bunch of beaming children always trailed behind her. It wasn't surprising. She pushed a standard hospital tea trolley, disguised as ' Willy Wonka's Chocolate Factory'. Every known type of sweet was displayed on the trolley. As well as sampling the wares, the children had the chance to distribute the sweets, in paper triangles, to other small patients too ill to leave their beds.

When she was up to it, Alice joined this happy procession in a wheelchair. Chloe pushed her along. This entitled both girls to a much-prized badge. 'Jolly Trolley' invariably asked Alice if she would help her with the Thursday evening run. Alice always did, except when she was too weak or racked with pain to rise. Then she would fret and ask her mother to apologise to 'Jolly Trolley'. 'Never mind,' said 'Jolly Trolley', 'there's another chance next week.' Alice never ate the sweets given to her by 'Jolly Trolley'; she just wanted to hand them out to cheer her fellow patients. It was another opportunity to show that she, and not her illness, was going to win this war.

* * *

As Alice waited eagerly for 'Jolly Trolley' night, Carol looked forward to the Tuesday evening visits of a female hospital chaplain. This hadn't always been true. When the woman introduced herself, Carol, until then a regular churchgoer, was struggling with her faith. Alice's sudden illness had given it a mighty knock. At first she did not welcome the chaplain at Alice's bedside. Afterwards, she was contrite and ashamed for snubbing this gentle woman. One day she did invite her over and the chaplain proved of considerable help in discussing the growing problem with Chloe.

Carol was becoming more aware of her older daughter's part in the drama they were all playing out. She suspected that Chloe was feeling left out; that Alice was getting all the love. Carol knew she was quite right to feel excluded; she felt guilty about lavishing most attention on her younger daughter. But what could she do? Alice needed her the most now. That was obvious. But how do you explain that to an eleven-year-old? The chaplain allowed Carol to talk freely about her guilt and together they explored ways to resolve the dilemma. 'I cried with her and she understood,' said Carol. 'She told me to take each problem and deal with it as it came up and to make time to reassure Chloe every time she seemed upset.'

Yet despite this sensible advice, Chloe continued to be a worry. She was not allowed to sleep in the ward, as Dean or Carol was, and every night she went home with Dean's mother. The whole of the summer holidays would be wasted by Alice's long stay in the hospital. Before the treatment became necessary, both girls had been promised all sorts of summer treats, such as days by the seaside, picnics and visits to theme parks. Denied these outings, Chloe complained bitterly to her mother. Slowly, she began to withdraw from the rest of the family. She started to whinge at every little thing and disobeyed her parents. Dean, not a natural disciplinarian, forced himself to be firm with her. He stopped asking her what she'd like to do, and instead started telling her. He reasoned that giving her choices was only confusing her. He also cut down on her visits to Alice.

Dean noticed Chloe was upset at seeing other patients. Two and a half years older than Alice, she was able to make more sense of the harrowing conversations around her. And she was horror-stricken to learn that many of the children on the ward would not live much longer. The schoolgirl was heartbroken by this. In hospital and at home she would suddenly break into tears both for Alice and her fellow patients. But though she was steadily withdrawing from her parents, her beatific nature would not allow her to desert her sister. On her less frequent visits to Ward 10, Chloe would read a story to Alice or just tell her what she'd been doing at home. If Alice were asleep, as she often was under the influence of her taxing treatments, Chloe would calmly lie by Alice's side, cuddling up to her on the bed. Dean and Carol were delighted to see that Chloe, despite feeling like the second favourite daughter, still had the strength to stay close to Alice. They were content to take the blame.

When Chloe visited Alice in hospital, she was always on the look out for children whose parents couldn't be there. She would sit with them, or help to colour a picture or bring them toys or a comic. The state of health of children in beds surrounding Alice was always on her mind. She was a member of the hospital's sibling group, a little club where brothers and sisters of the sick children talk and play together, under the watchful eye of social workers and play therapists.

The sad story of one young member of this little band was always on Chloe's mind. She often talks about it, never without tears, 'There was this girl in our group. She was called Amy and she had long blonde hair and blue eyes. And she always wore a cap. She was about twelve. She had a sister who was seven. They had a brother whom she said was lovely. He had a brain tumour.

'She said she'd stayed by his bedside, while he just lay there. She loved him a lot. He never moved. Then he died. And she even stayed and talked to him when he was dead. He was still lying on his bed and she couldn't stop talking because she loved him so much. She said she was very sad, but she said she didn't cry because she wanted to be brave for her sister. 'She told me her brother had wanted to be a fireman when he grew older. She said four firemen carried his little coffin at the funeral. It was very sad.'

* * *

It's a heartbreaking fact that, despite all the efforts of tireless and extremely skilful staff, many children on Ward 10 will die. One day, on the way out after visiting Alice, her grandfather Harry met an expensively dressed consultant he'd not seen before. He told him how heartened he was to see so many children, many without hair, playing happily between the beds, seemingly without a care in the world. 'Yes,' agreed the doctor sorrowfully, 'and it's a shame that six out of ten of them will not survive.' A few minutes later, Harry shared the lift to the ground floor with a young man who looked very unkempt and dirty. A smart dresser himself, he looked at his fellow passenger curiously. The man must have sensed an air of disapproval because he said suddenly, 'My child is very ill and needs me all the time now. I haven't had a chance to wash or shave for two weeks. I've not eaten properly either.' Harry felt sorry for judging the man so hastily. He wept on the way home.

Dean and Carol were also becoming ashamed of some of their feelings on the ward. Though the couple were irritated with other parents because they so often seemed humourless and defeated, they gradually came to wonder if they were being intolerant and unfair. After all, many families were suffering more than they were. Most had been coming to Ward 10 for longer than the Maddocks. And they were trying to hold down jobs with less flexible hours. Some had to take work all through the night, just to be with their poorly child during the day. Often a mother would visit all through the daylight hours – to be replaced by a sleepy dad at night, or the other way round.

Even Alice's parents, with their understanding bosses, had difficulty squeezing everything in. Occasionally either Dean or Carol came home to spend precious time with Chloe and do household chores, like ironing and catching up with the post. This was regarded as a treat, because they were 'normal', as opposed to their unnatural life on the ward. 'It was so lovely to come back occasionally,' said Dean, 'and have egg and chips. To enjoy sitting down with no noise, to be able to slump in front of the telly, with nobody choosing what we had to watch.'

The colony of television sets on the ward was a menace. The Maddocks found themselves hearing, without listening, to the worst of morning, afternoon and evening programmes round the clock. 'When you're caring for your very sick child, worrying all the time, the last thing you want is smirking television people with their false cheerfulness,' said Carol. 'Most of the time we felt like picking up the nearest TV set and chucking it through the window.' When they wanted to watch the odd programme themselves, Dean and Carol used earphones provided by the hospital. But few of the other parents bothered. They just turned the volume up.

When the family first came onto the ward they were surprised that parents aired so many whinges about the facilities, food and furnishings. It seemed so petty and ungrateful, given the seriousness of their children's conditions and the hard work of the staff. But soon the Maddocks recognized that many of the complaints were justified. Expecting children to live in such tired, shabby inadequate surroundings was not on – and it was worth complaining about.

Alice refused all the hospital meals that came round on trolleys, other than cereal with cold milk for breakfast. Carol couldn't blame her. On offer were chips, strong smelling boiled cabbage, lumpy mashed potato and sago pudding served on plastic plates. Her parents were obliged to provide Alice with their own alternatives. Dean spent hours in the confined kitchen, making pasta with fresh salad and sandwiches. In between, Alice nibbled on cheese strings, cherry tomatoes and biscuits.

Poor surroundings led to frayed tempers. Nurses and doctors had to put up with streams of abuse about the lack of facilities. Side wards were highly prized, and parents would often harangue or even threaten staff to try and get one for their child. They would also argue with other parents in heated exchanges, laced with obscenities. Dean remembers a fight, which broke out about midnight. One mother thumped another for some reason he never discovered. The indignant victim rained more blows in return and outraged nurses had to separate them.

The family would have been happy to put up with all the indignities on Ward 10 if they knew that Alice's treatment would lengthen her life. But the doctors gave no guarantees. They admitted that it was all trial and error. And if this treatment wasn't effective, then they would have to alter the regime slightly and try again. That meant poor Alice might need to keep coming back to Ward 10 time and time again.

* * *

During this sombre period, an angel came to the bedside and kept on coming. She was Tracey Booth-Gibbons, a neighbour and a midwife at St James's. She used to arrive either at the end or the beginning of her shift, or on rare days off. When Alice is at home, she plays with Tracey's six-year-old Olivia and Luke who's in her class at school. This bubbly, down-to-earth visitor, a dear friend of the family, is no stranger to childhood tragedy. Her first baby girl, Amy, had breathing difficulties, possibly caused by a virus and died sixteen days after being born. Another infant, Sam, had major problems with his circulation and didn't survive birth.

'With some visitors it could be a bit of a strain talking,' said Carol, 'but, perhaps because of what had happened to her children, Tracey knew exactly what we were going through. She just sat there quietly – or she would gently talk to me – and I became calm.' Carol spent many hours with Tracey in the months ahead and she would endlessly discuss what was best for Alice and Chloe. Carol would confide in Tracey and they had long discussions about the possibility of having another child. Another child might give them the perfect match for Alice. This was something Dean and Carol had given great thought to, but was it right to bring another child into the world to be used to save Alice?

Eventually the day came when Alice's treatment, which had seemed never ending, did come to a close. Six weeks after Alice first entered the hospital gates the family was told she could go home. Everybody was thrilled. The drive back to their home was joyous and carefree. They plumped down in the living room with sighs of happiness. Soon Alice's hefty bundle of get-well cards was stuck on the living room walls with Blu-tack, as a reminder of the loving support of family and friends. But sadly the pure glee of being together again in their cosy home wasn't to last. After a few brief hours, something frightening befell Alice. Something very frightening indeed...

Serum Sickness

Alice's first night at home brought a nasty surprise. It looked very much as if serum sickness was setting in. This is a much-feared reaction to the very toxic immunosuppression treatment she'd just completed at St James's. Put simply, Alice's body was trying to reject the foreign agents introduced into her blood. The little girl woke up just before midnight complaining of bothersome pins and needles in her feet. Dean and Carol stayed up with her till she fell asleep again at 5 a.m. By 8.30 a.m., Alice's temperature had climbed nearly 2°C to 38.4°C, a serious change for a patient with a weakened immune system. (The normal body temperature for a girl of Alice's age is 36.5°C.) Half an hour later, the mercury was still climbing. Alice felt sick. There was a reddish rash spreading across her face and chest.

Doctors at St James's were consulted on the phone. They were sceptical that this was a case of serum sickness, but arranged that

Alice should return to Ward 10 anyway, in case she'd picked up some sort of infection. Within an hour of Dean making that call, a muddled and very poorly Alice was back in hospital. Her temperature was now abnormally high at 38.9°C.

Despite the severity of her symptoms, hospital staff still doubted Alice actually had serum sickness. That was because this scourge usually kicks in one to three weeks after treatment, not the next day. The consensus remained that Alice had picked up some kind of hospital infection. To bring down Alice's lofty temperature, nurses dosed her with paracetamol, a painkiller and anti-fever agent, and Piriton, a drug to treat allergic reactions. They gave her anti-sickness agents and steroids. Her arm was connected to a bedside drip to stop her becoming dehydrated. All these measures helped – for the time being – and Alice slept better than the previous night. In the morning, she was playing again with six-month-old Nisa, who was still in the same cot. But later in the day Alice couldn't play with anyone...

The following day she looked tired and drawn. Her hair seemed dull and lifeless. There were bluish smudges under her eyes and dark hollows in her cheeks. She was off her food. An angry red rash enveloped both legs. Soon, her limbs looked as though they'd been dipped in boiling tar. The skin itched mercilessly and was covered in angry purple bruises.

Going to the toilet with her distraught father, she felt sharp pains attack her groin. It was becoming hard to walk. Her legs were slowly stiffening. Both knees were starting to hurt. A short tour of the ward in a vain bid to get rid of the stiffness ended when Dean had to pick up his daughter and carry her back to bed. He thought she looked really ill now, her eyes exaggerated by fever. A nurse was called and noted that her temperature had soared to a raging 39.5°C. Her pulse raced at 170 per minute, compared to the normal rate of 110. Dean knew very little about serum sickness, but he doubted Alice's terrifying symptoms had anything to do with a common infection. Carol had already boned up on serum sickness and fearfully identified the same signs in Alice. She had also frightened herself by reading that there was no effective means of stopping the symptoms spreading.

The little girl was obviously getting worse. She could hardly move at all now. Her neck, shoulders, elbows, wrists, hips and legs – in fact, every joint in her slender body – were all seizing up. Her fingers and toes had swollen like sausages. She was burning, fiery hot, yet her hands and feet were icy cold.

Carol keeps an occasional diary. For that day, she penned, 'Alice is screaming in pain...screaming...it's horrible to see her in such torment.'

A doctor, disturbed at Alice's deteriorating condition, injected morphine. Her parents waited anxiously. That was better. Within minutes the agony had eased slightly. Carol and Dean asked a doctor why the pain had been so severe. He explained that the torment resulted from bone rubbing against bone. The powerful drugs of the anti-immune treatment had had a draconian effect. They'd dissolved away the soft ligament between the joints of Alice's bones. There was now nothing left to separate and cushion them. Ultra-sensitive nerve endings were scraping and rasping together.

'I felt like crying, no, screaming, at the thought of my baby going through this dreadful pain,' said Carol. She also agonised yet again over whether they'd been right to allow the anti-immune treatment to go ahead at all. They'd brought a child who was healthy and carefree into hospital – and now look at her. She was in a piteous state, racked by vehement pain, sometimes lifeless and completely stiff. Her normally clear skin was now purple, angry and blistered. She was in agony.

* * *

The couple noticed a certain lack of direction in the treatment of their daughter. They were troubled to learn from the staff that indeed there was no set treatment for Alice's appalling symptoms. Every case was different and the doctors were forced to rely on trial and error. By now Carol was beside herself with worry. 'Alice was in a deplorable state. Her blood pressure, pulse and her breathing were all off the wall. And none of these problems seemed the least bit improved by the drugs they were giving her.'

Alice wasn't the only child suffering on Ward 10. A little girl in the bed next to hers went into anaphylactic shock. This causes the body to shut down almost completely, rather like switching off a robot. The child very nearly died. Carol realised, to her horror, that her symptoms were very similar to Alice's. And then she noticed that the child's parents were scrutinising Alice's every move with fearful eyes.

Despite her intense suffering, Alice was still unnerved by people who couldn't help staring at her. Rather than be watched, she always refused a bedpan. As she wouldn't use a wheelchair either, Dean had to constantly carry her to the toilet. Careful though he was not to jar her, this would cause Alice to screech out in pain, screams that echoed down the long ward. 'Shrieks like you've never heard before,' observed Carol grimly. 'They were deafening. And that horrifying sound was coming from our darling Alice, putting up with searing pain.'

Both Dean and Carol thought their younger daughter would not live for long now. Carol entreated nurses to find Alice a side ward, for her sake and for the sake of other children who were frightened by her piercing shouts of agony. Eventually a little girl, suffering from leukaemia, was moved from a side ward into the main area so that Alice could take her place. Unbeknown to Dean or Carol, that young patient was Molly-Ann Barnett, who was later to make headline news all over the world, and change the life of the Maddocks family forever...

With their new privacy in the side ward came an immense feeling of relief. No more prying eyes. No strangers looking on. The three of them, and Chloe on her frequent visits, could be themselves again, with nobody to judge their reactions to Alice's illness or ask questions about her. Even so, Dean felt uncomfortable about the importance he attached to this privacy. Alice was bearing indescribable agonies caused by her body's grotesque revenge against drugs added to her system. Yet Dean and his wife were irritated that everyone could hear Alice's cries of pain and witness her parents' distress. It was as if Alice's suffering was embarrassing them. This seemed a trivial response considering what was at stake.

The distraught pair did all they could to keep Alice comfortable. 'We bathed her forehead and spoke soothing words. We laid cold wet towels across her fevered little chest,' Dean recalls. But they felt, and actually were, helpless in the face of such relentless suffering. The serum sickness showed no sign of waning. In fact, if anything, its hideous symptoms were becoming even worse. A glum-faced, kindly consultant came one day and warned them that Alice was seriously ill and that this suffering might only be the beginning. More frighteningly, he added that they must now 'be prepared to lose Alice at almost any time'. He bleakly warned them, 'You must treasure every moment – as every day is a bonus with serum sickness.'

* * *

Dean was in no doubt, though he didn't confide in Carol, that they had just been prepared for the moment when their beloved daughter would pass away. *'Be prepared to lose Alice at almost any time.'* The words engraved themselves on Carol's mind. 'I felt so tired, mentally and physically, because we'd gone nights with barely any sleep and now the worst was happening. I knew I had to cope but wondered how I'd get the strength to do so.'

Alice was suffering the severe side effects of a drastic treatment, a backlash that would probably kill her. This news, given gently and gravely, was a deep shock for the parents. Carol slipped quietly away to the toilet, 'I got down on my knees behind a cubicle door and began praying. "Please God, don't take Alice from us," I begged over and over again. I wanted Alice to have her childhood back, to watch her enjoy school, then go to university, to grow up into a lovely mature young lady. I wanted her to be as happy as she used to be. I prayed on that ghastly, grotty, smelly toilet floor, asking God to give us another chance, not to take Alice away. But if that had to be, and she had to die, that He would give us the strength we needed to deal with it.'

Carol wanted to be rid of her feelings of guilt, brought about by her own illness when Alice was born. Kneeling in that small, dingy cubicle was a world away from 5 September 1992, the day Alice Rose Maddocks entered the world three weeks earlier than she should have. Weighing 6lb 3oz, with tufts of dark brown hair, Alice was a pretty baby. But within two weeks of that day, Carol began suffering severe postnatal depression, which continued for many months.

During this difficult time she could not bond with Alice and found it hard to provide the most basic care for her tiny baby.

'I felt I was now being punished for this, paying the price for those dark days and I was wracked with guilt. I know it is untrue and irrational but at the time, I hated myself and felt I was a bad, undeserving mother,' Carol recalls. 'It took me some months before I could understand some logic into the illness I suffered and accept that it wasn't linked to Alice's condition.'

That night, neither parent slept as they kept vigil over their gravely ill daughter. For every minute the awful phrase assailed their overactive minds: *'Be prepared to lose Alice at almost any time.'* Because of her swollen joints, she couldn't move. If she managed by a huge effort to change position, she stayed like that for hours on end. The inside of her mouth was scratched and parched and sore, her lips cracked. She itched all over. Even the inside of her eyelids itched. But she was unable to scratch anywhere, as her swollen hands and arms wouldn't obey her. When Carol and Dean tried to scratch for her, they saw purple bruises breaking through her chalky white skin. They spent hour after hour trying to cool down her burning flesh with more damp flannels, occasionally applying calamine lotion. But nothing seemed to stop the unnaturally intense itching. *'Be prepared to lose Alice at almost any time.'*

Her skin was also blistering as if a malevolent spirit were applying an invisible blowtorch. Carol thought she looked like a child, who'd just been through a nuclear war, as though she'd been burnt by radiation. And she could almost see her shedding weight. To ease the constant pain, Alice was given regular injections of morphine. Afterwards she lay inert with her eyes closed, spent, utterly lifeless. She was a broken doll.

Not sure whether she could hear or not, Carol or Dean read her long stories. When they finally put down the book, though Alice seemed comatose, she always mouthed, though didn't say, 'thank you'. For long hours, Dean imagined his daughter was walking on very thin ice. Any moment she might slip through the surface and her life would cease.

* * *

Then, after 25 hours of incessant suffering that both parents will never forget, in all its hideous detail, Alice's condition began to stabilise. Her parents watched carefully, hardly daring to breathe. Small hopeful signs began to show. Soon Carol was able to add to her diary, 'Alice had a much better night. She's still in a great deal of pain, but it's now under control.' One by one, her dreadful symptoms slowly subsided. The last side effect to disappear was the stiffness in her knees. The serum sickness was spent. The staff on Ward 10 were surprised that Alice had recovered so quickly. It wouldn't be the last time that Alice's restorative powers were to amaze the doctors treating her.

There was, however, one hiccup in the recovery process. The day came when they were asked to forfeit their precious side ward for a more urgent case. The thought of strangers watching her in bed frightened Alice so much that an odd thing happened to her voice. As she was about to move back into the main ward, she regressed to the speech patterns of a toddler. She clung to her parents like a shy two-year-old. This odd behaviour moved Dean to implore the hospital authorities to change their minds. But it was no use; Alice had to return to the main ward. Alice bitterly blamed her parents for losing her private retreat. This was the peevish, petulant side of their child they already knew about, but rarely saw.

A Brief Encounter

One night, as Alice continued to shrug off serum sickness, Carol was walking back from the kitchen, down the corridor towards Alice's bed, when she saw a tall, slim woman, four or five years older than herself, coming the other way. Carol recognised the care-worn expression of a parent in the same boat as herself. She wore the same strangely vacant, distracted look of a mother with a seriously ill child, at odds with her smart clothes. Carol thought, 'I know how she feels; you can't look after your own health when you care for your sick child.' The stranger smiled and asked, 'Hello, are you new?' She introduced herself as Mandy Barnett, the mother of the little girl who'd given up her side ward for Alice.

Mandy and Carol were to become firm friends. At that time, Molly-Ann was dangerously ill with acute leukaemia, and her parents were involved in a strenuous campaign to recruit bone marrow donors to save her life. Carol was unaware of this battle, until Mandy asked her if they too were searching for a donor for Alice. 'What do you mean?' she responded. 'Isn't finding a donor up to "Dr Mike"?'

'Well, if they find a match for Alice out of the few donors available, you'll be very lucky.'

Carol was stunned. She'd never imagined that the right kind of bone marrow wasn't freely available. She stammered, 'But I thought it was just there, waiting on a shelf.' She was too troubled to carry on the conversation and she couldn't wait to leave Mandy. A cold hand seized her heart. She was struck by the awful realisation that finding a donor for Alice wasn't going to be as easy as they'd thought. Other panicky thoughts tumbled through her head. People were giving blood all the time, weren't they? Anybody who needed it could get it. It must be the same with bone marrow. Mustn't it? Come to think of it, though she knew people who gave blood, including Dean, she'd never met anyone who donated marrow. Why were people not queuing up to give bone marrow? She and Dean had always thought the procedure was as simple as giving blood. But now it seemed it wasn't. It was beginning to look as though Alice's life was again hanging on a thread.

While these reflections turned Carol's face pale and her skin clammy, Mandy Barnett was asking if Alice had lost her hair. 'No,' said Carol, distractedly 'It's a different treatment to the one given for leukaemia. But Alice is still terrified that she'll soon go bald.' Mandy sympathised and invited Alice to meet Molly-Ann in her hospital bed. Molly-Ann's long straw-coloured hair had been temporarily sacrificed to chemotherapy. Mandy reasoned that if

Alice could talk to a patient of her own age, with similar interests, then she'd quickly conquer her fear.

However, the meeting was postponed until Molly-Ann had recovered from an infection that made her eyes swollen and discoloured. As it happened, the two little girls never met in hospital. But it was this chance encounter with Molly-Ann's mother that sparked a whirlwind of events which brought Alice to world-wide attention – and which eventually gave thousands of children and adults a new chance of life.

* * *

Alice was discharged at the beginning of September. She was still in pain, severe enough to need regular doses of morphine. While it was true the drugs she'd taken had successfully subdued her immune system, preventing it from destroying her bone marrow, her severely weakened body carried a new danger. She was largely unprotected from invading germs, including pneumonia, tuberculosis and meningitis. All these diseases would be even worse than normal if Alice were exposed to them. A dose of flu could be fatal and an attack of conjunctivitis could cause blindness. A heavy course of antibiotics was prescribed to try to protect her against potentially fatal bugs like these. She was also being given steroids. In fact, the family returned home with a vast collection of pills and potions, together with a complex timetable of when they should be given.

Very early in her illness, even before anyone knew Alice had a fault in her bone marrow, she'd started to perspire heavily at night. Carol put this down to bad dreams. But once the effects of serum sickness were behind her, Alice started sweating again. The Maddocks learned later that this was due to the body's struggle to make her bone marrow work properly again. It was just one more indignity the proud little girl had to suffer.

The only true consolation during Alice's suffering was that Dean and Carol knew she was in excellent hands. Their confidence in 'Dr Mike' grew month by month. If they had to wait two hours after their appointment time to see him, that was because he gave a lot of time to talking to his patients. Dean said, 'He'll answer any little question with great patience. We never felt he was pushing us towards the door. Our respect for him just grew by the minute and we gradually came to trust him completely with Alice's life.'

* * *

Though many parents around her had given up on their personal appearance to care for their sick child, Carol strove hard to look clean and tidy. She had a shower every day, never forgot her make-up and tried daily to find a different outfit. 'I didn't feel like doing any of this, but I didn't want people to think things were getting on top of us,' she explained. 'And I needed Alice to feel nothing had changed. If we let ourselves go, then she would worry that something was really wrong. We didn't want her to know that was true.'

Even when she was suffering most, Carol tried to make Alice look her best. She bought her a new toilet bag and filled it with her soap, flannel, shampoo, toothbrush and toothpaste. She gave her a bed bath every morning, dressed her with fresh clothes and even varnished her nails. Sometimes Alice was well enough to appreciate this ritual; sometimes she was too poorly to care. As her health improved, Alice would point out other children on the ward and insist that her mother do their nails, too. Dean pitched in by helping Alice make mobiles to hang over her bed. He wanted to make Alice's hospital bed space as much like her own room as possible.

Carol said, 'We both worked so hard to make Alice feel at home. Because it was only now, when we feared losing her, that we realised just how precious she was. When I gave birth, I just took it for granted that she was ours forever, that I would see her finish school, travel, become a mum and now I was coming to know this isn't guaranteed, not with Alice, not with any child.'

In odd moments by the bedside, Carol searched for a reason why God had allowed Alice to develop this awful condition. Surely, He wouldn't put Alice through such an ordeal if it weren't for a very good purpose. She now believes Alice's illness was brought about by divine forces to enlarge the bone marrow register and save thousands of lives. This conviction, born as Alice suffered her worst in hospital, explains why the family was able to endure so much pain and humiliation over the coming months ...

The Christmas Present

On the day they left St James's for the second time, in November 2000, Alice refused to go home straight away. She planned to find a toyshop. So they called at a nearby shopping centre. There, Dean spotted a store that sold and rented wheelchairs. In hospital, Alice hadn't objected to being trundled around on wheels. This was a relief to her parents because the pains and cramps in her legs and knees meant she couldn't walk or even stand for more than a few moments. While Alice chose a toy, Dean called at the shop alone and hired a wheelchair as a surprise. But when he pushed it towards her, Alice astonished him by freezing in disgust. She refused even to look at it. Inside the hospital and within its grounds were appropriate places for a wheelchair, but her young pride wouldn't allow its use under watchful eyes in the street.

Although Alice was still feeling weak and floppy, she walked gamely with her parents around the shopping centre for over an hour. Behind her, Dean, now bitterly regretting his impulse, shoved the empty chair. Alice even offered to push it round for him at one point. But it was all a show. 'She was still in so much pain,' said Dean. 'Her legs were cramping up, again. She was leaning on me and on Carol. She would sit on the edge of displays in shops, prop herself up in doorways, anything for a bit of a rest. She was grey and perspiring with effort. She was trying so hard to show us she was well again – that she could do anything we could. Like her mother, Alice never, ever gives up.'

The couple were soon made aware that Alice was not just physically affected by severe aplastic anaemia. She was now battling with insecurity. The first sign was that she became frightened of her own bedroom. Perhaps it was because sefrum sickness had first surfaced there. At any event, on their first evening back at home, Alice simply refused to sleep in the room. Dean tried to be firm, but she would get out of bed at every opportunity and ramble all over the house in the night. Carol tried to allay Alice's fears by lying on her bed with her, until she fell asleep. Naturally, an exhausted Carol would also doze off, waking up hours later, stiff-necked and irritable. Exasperated, Dean considered redecorating the bedroom, but had neither the time to do it himself nor the money to pay somebody else.

In the end, the only way out of the problem was to allow a victorious Alice to sleep between her parents. The steroids Alice was taking caused the main drawback to this arrangement. They boosted her appetite, causing her to wake several times in the night and, like a cuckoo in a nest, demand feeding. Her list of requirements included cheese strings, chicken, corned beef sandwiches and rice pudding.

* * *

Still, things could have been worse. Alice was back at school, Dean and Carol were working again and everyone agreed the little girl's eccentric behaviour was better than life in hospital.

The autumn had passed with Alice in relatively good health. With Christmas in sight, the family had their first good news since Alice went sprawling in her school friend's garden at the beginning of the summer. It came when Carol took Alice to St James's for one of her routine transfusions. She wasn't expecting to see 'Dr Mike' that day, but he sought them out to tell them something wonderful.

'We've been looking at the registers and I'm pleased to tell you there are 35 possible matches for Alice.'

Carol froze. Then her face turned white with joy. 'This was it! This was it! I was ecstatic. I wasn't over the moon, but the furthest star! Obviously, there was going to be at least one ideal donor is such a long list. This was it! We had found our donor.'

She only just stopped herself hugging 'Dr Mike'. Instead, she embraced her daughter in a long tight hug. Alice burrowed into her. 'We just might have a donor, Alice. A donor.' Carol knew not to overreact, but this was the best news yet.

The consultant spoke calmly, gently warning them that tests were still needed on the 35 samples to check for an exact tissue type. It would still take a few weeks to be absolutely sure.

But Carol wouldn't be discouraged. Good grief, she thought again, out of three dozen lovely people, there must be at least one perfect donor, probably more than one. She left Alice in a pile of hospital toys and rushed outside, reaching for her mobile phone. The sky was a dark, pinky yellow. Snow was drifting down quite heavily, like shredded ticker tape at a victory parade. Despite the cold cottony flakes on her cheeks, there was sun in Carol's heart as she phoned Dean. She couldn't savour the whole of his delighted reaction, because she hung up on him and began calling nearly everyone she knew. Mother Nature spread icing on the tarmac as her message went out to a dozen homes – 'Alice is safe.'

'Anybody who saw me in those hospital grounds would think I'd won millions on the pools. A miracle had just taken place. We'd been given back Alice's life.'

On a wave of happiness, Carol and Dean prepared to give the girls the best Christmas ever.

The Sky Falls in Again

At least the disappointment came on them slowly. But it was still a heavy cross to bear. Slowly, one by one, the names were whittled down. Finally, every one of the 35 potential donors had been ruled out. A few of the volunteers had moved and couldn't be traced. Two were no longer healthy enough to give marrow safely. Three others were a very near match, but not near enough and so on.

Dean and Carol were utterly crestfallen. What a letdown! After expecting their daughter to make a full recovery, Dean and Carol were now learning the true difficulty of finding anyone who could supply the much-needed marrow. Not only was Alice's tissue type proving very rare indeed, but they'd discovered another peril: the bone marrow registers were unreliable. This was hard to bear.

Of the 350,000 names on the Anthony Nolan list – the biggest of the British bone marrow registers – how many were actually valid? If four or five out of the 35 near matches chosen for Alice were unsuitable or unavailable, wasn't it likely that thousands of people on the full list would be useless as well? So not only did the Maddocks have to bear the crushing disappointment that their 35 possible donors couldn't help after all, but they'd now lost all confidence in the registration system.

'We'd never felt so miserable,' said Dean.

The Searchers

It was now clear that the first course of immunosuppressive drug treatment had not put Alice into remission and she was dependent on weekly transfusions of blood and platelets to keep her alive. The couple had a choice: they could either sit around hoping the hospital would eventually find that perfect donor, or they could shorten the odds by campaigning themselves for more volunteers. Of course, they picked the more active option.

They would begin by adding their own names to the bone marrow registers. Fine – but how to go about it? They didn't know who to contact. Dean had given blood for fifteen years, but nobody had ever told him that he could also donate his bone marrow – never mind how to do it. 'I'd never seen any posters about bone marrow or picked up a leaflet,' he said, 'which is odd, because you do read everything you lay your eyes on during those long blood-giving sessions.' Once again, the couple consulted the Internet, where they learned all they needed to know.

Then for step two – persuading other people to sign up. A friend of Dean's brother ran off a few posters on a computer. It had a picture of Alice, with a short definition of severe aplastic anaemia.

There was an explanation of why she needed a donor and how to give bone marrow through the National Blood Service or the Anthony Nolan Trust.

One of Dean's initial aims – and one which the couple continue to push now – is that people who come to donate blood should, at the same time, give a second blood sample with a view to providing bone marrow. As far as he knew this was not being done, though it must be easy enough to arrange. He turned his attention to the Anthony Nolan Trust. This was a charity set up many years ago by Shirley Nolan OBE, after her small son Anthony had died for want of a suitable donor. This charity maintains its own register of donors.

Surely this well-known body would welcome the idea of asking blood donors to go one step further with their bone marrow. But again Dean was disappointed. It seemed that the Anthony Nolan Trust had recently changed its rules, actually making it harder for bone marrow donors to sign up. Before this policy change, the Trust organised clinics in the name of a local patient in need of a bone marrow transplant. People who came along were asked to give a tiny blood sample. From this, analysts worked out their bone marrow group and added their details to the national register.

It sounded like a sensible, foolproof system. But it wasn't. There'd been serious problems. People would come to the clinics to help one specific friend or relative who needed a bone marrow transplant. But when they found their details would be added to a national register to help strangers, they would make excuses and vanish. Or worse, they would ring up the Anthony Nolan Trust weeks later and ask for their names to be deleted from the list.

When Dean offered to organise new clinics in Alice's name to sample more donors, the Anthony Nolan Trust turned the idea down. Instead, they suggested Dean and Carol should organise a few 'information evenings'. The thinking behind these events was that people who came along would hear a speech from a Trust representative on exactly what was involved. They could then go away, read the leaflets, think it over – and if they were still happy, sign up through their own doctor. Dean thought all this palaver would put donors off.

He was also depressed to discover that the Anthony Nolan Trust was short of funds. And this was a big drawback, because it's not cheap to take blood samples, process them and add names to the list. In fact, it costs £50 per volunteer. This includes doctors' fees, analysing blood types and paperwork. Another disturbing discovery was that the government's own National Blood Service depended on yet another charity, called the British Bone Marrow Donor Appeal, to supply them with £250,000 a year. A vital NHS service relying on charity? That didn't seem at all right.

To the couple, both the National Blood Service and the Anthony Nolan Trust seemed in a weak position to save Alice's life – and those of hundreds of other children. But, of course, the Trust and the Blood Service argue that they are merely protecting patients from distressing problems that long experience has taught them to avoid.

* * *

It all seemed rather a nightmare to the Maddocks. And it wasn't going to be easy to put things right. They even found it difficult to recruit other parents to their cause, because most of them confidently believed the registers would produce the right donor for their child, sooner rather than later. It was this gap – between the cold reality of the sparse registers and the high expectations of parents – that Carol and Dean were destined to close. And, though they could never have imagined it at this early stage, they were soon to recruit the most powerful man in Britain to help them do it.

But for now, the couple spent hours round the kitchen table puzzling out how they could give Alice the chance of life. One of their early ploys was to write to the newspapers. This letter, from *The Mail on Sunday*, is one of dozens published when their campaign was in its infancy:

We have a happy daughter called Alice who may die. In the last twelve months, only 18,000 people joined the Bone Marrow Register – only achieved by families campaigning for their loved ones. There are many hundreds whose lives are now at serious risk. Please help us. We're desperate! – Dean and Carol Maddocks.

Each letter sent to a newspaper produced a new flood of emails from more people wanting to offer their bone marrow and sympathetic editors nearly always included Alice's website address.

Soon the dynamic duo refined their crusade with an attack on those controlling the government's register. They wrote to leaders of the National Blood Service in Yorkshire. Their letter asked if someone could explain why, when the couple were so anxious to find more donors by organising their own clinics, barriers were raised against them. In reply, they were invited to meet officials at the National Blood Service's regional headquarters in Seacroft Hospital, Leeds. This was promising. Perhaps at last somebody in authority was taking notice.

They went to the hospital expecting a warm welcome for their ideas and zeal. But their suggestions were doused in cold water. Senior staff confided that if more volunteers came forward, they wouldn't be able to cope with the extra workload. They revealed that samples from would-be donors were already overflowing their freezers. There weren't enough resources to process them. Carol wasn't satisfied with this. If there were difficulties, she thought bitterly, they shouldn't be making excuses. They should be launching an all-out effort to overcome them.

At that time the National Blood Service had two million blood donors on its books, yet the tally of names on their bone marrow register stood at a mere 100,000. Surely, Carol told the meeting, at least half of those blood-givers – presumably all caring people – would be happy to give marrow, too. But that didn't cut any ice; she was getting nowhere.

The afternoon dragged on without concessions. Glancing at his watch, Dean determined to salvage what he could from the meeting. He asked politely why there were no 'Be a Bone Marrow Donor' posters on the walls at blood donation sessions. Why no leaflets, either? He even offered to make and supply posters to the service. 'But I'm not sure they wanted to know,' he bemoaned afterwards.

The couple acknowledged that sometimes 'bone marrow' leaflets were left lying about for people who'd already given blood and were having tea and biscuits. But why weren't they handed out beforehand? Then a sample could be taken for bone marrow analysis on the same visit. Dean told the meeting, 'What's happening all over the country is that people are picking up a leaflet as they leave the clinic, only to abandon it unread in the glove compartment.'

However, the encounter in Seacroft Hospital ended on a higher note when officials promised to raise all the Maddocks' ideas at their next regional meeting. 'Fair enough,' thought Dean optimistically. 'They'll all come round to our view when they've thought it over properly.'

But the regional big wigs surprised him again. They wrote back to say they would make no changes as they were already doing all they could to find a donor for Alice. Dean and Carol were hurt and angry. They knew for a fact that the official objective for new bone marrow donors was only 5,000 a year – and that was not a local target, but a national one. How could that be 'doing everything'?

The gloves were off now! Alice would never be saved this way! The couple vowed not to allow staff of the National Blood Service any peace. They involved themselves in long conversations and arguments with officials at every opportunity for months ahead, pressing them to greater efforts. But the local service wouldn't officially admit to a shortage of resources, never mind do anything about it.

Plainly, more drastic action was called for – and the Maddocks went under cover...

The Blood Spies

Obstructed by officialdom from organising their own donor sessions, the intrepid couple turned suspicious eyes on official blood sessions held all over West Yorkshire. They found themselves doing a Sherlock Holmes on the service. Travelling many miles, Dean and

Carol clandestinely visited the clinics to check if any 'bone marrow' leaflets or posters were on display. Usually, they weren't. Wearing inconspicuous drab clothing, spectacles with dirty lenses and trying to look insignificant, they sidled up to donors sitting in the clinics and listened keenly to see if staff offered advice on how to give bone marrow. They rarely did. With overcoat collars upturned, Dean and Carol lurked outside, asking people who'd just given blood if they'd seen bone marrow literature or posters inside. Few of them had.

Sometimes working separately but usually together, the couple did their spying undetected for some time. But in due course they were recognised. This had some interesting effects. Staff would suddenly cease chatting together and move away from the couple, or they would talk loudly about the benefits of bone marrow donation in their presence. Occasionally they spotted red-faced staff fishing around in battered boxes under tables in a bit of a dither. They were evidently hunting for hidden sheaves of leaflets to hurriedly display in a prominent position.

Dean and Carol were pleased to find there were 'moles' within the ranks. Evidently not everybody in the National Blood Service was wary of the couple. They began to collect a few smiles and words of encouragement from the staff at clinics. A few pats on the back were given. One day someone quietly handed Dean a complete list of all new donor sessions in the north of England – at church halls, community centres, small factories and so on. This 'hit list' proved extremely useful.

Dean posted a pack of posters to all the venues on this 'leaked' schedule. Each one bore a photo of Alice in her Brownie uniform. His covering letter proclaimed, 'The Blood Service won't advertise for bone marrow, so will you please put these posters up?' He hoped that the person running the session, a caretaker, a vicar or business manager, say, would sympathise with Alice's plight and do what was asked. He was rarely disappointed. Letters came back saying the posters had been tacked up in prominent places and wishing Alice the best of luck.

But even with this sort of help, the covert publicity campaign was tough going. First they had to compile the posters on their computer

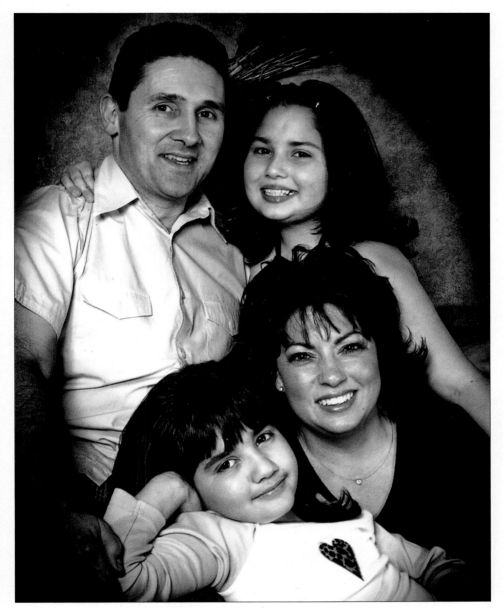

The battling Maddocks – Dean, Carol, Chloe and Alice – a loving family bound even closer together by a rare and dangerous illness.

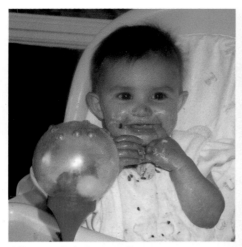

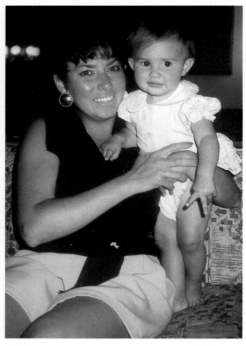

Alice, aged eleven months.

Happier times: Carol with Alice when she was twelve months old (right).

Below: Five-year-old Alice on her first day at school with Chloe, aged eight.

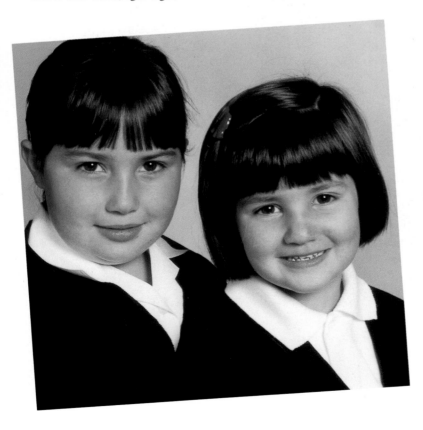

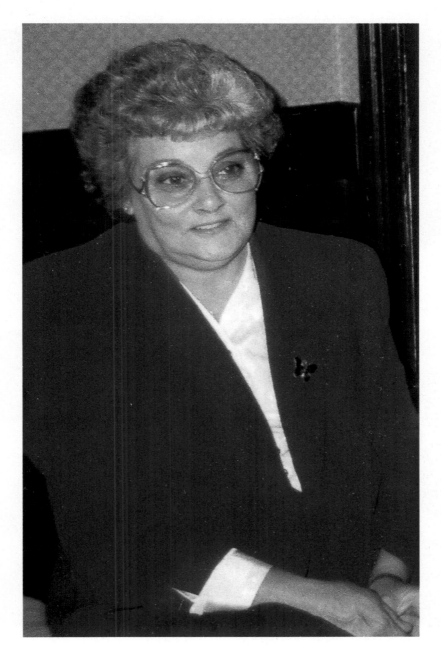

Carol's late mother, Pat, who seemed to warn her daughter through a dream that Alice would soon be in danger. Carol says she's inherited her mum's fighting spirit.

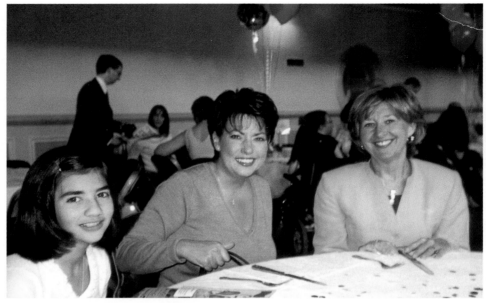

Alice, Carol and head teacher Bev Drury, who's astonished at the sure way her valiant pupil copes with such a serious illness.

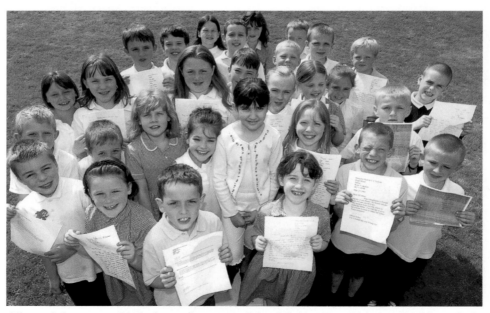

Alice and classmates with the letters they sent to Prime Minister Tony Blair, begging him to find more money in the hunt for a bone marrow donor.

Opposite: One of the letters from Alice's school friends to Tony Blair. They were all bundled up and sent to Downing Street.

Monday 21st May.

Dear. Mr. Blair
        I ame writing
about my Frend Alice Maddocks
She has. got servere Aplastic
A reamia. She can not play out
or do P.E. The school would
love Alice to get better. I think
what Alice dose for us. She would
like Alice to get belter soon
        Your sincerely
        Timothy

Alice Needs YOU

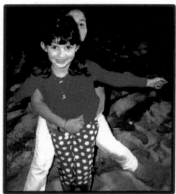

This is Alice, our lovely eight-year-old daughter. She has a condition known as "Severe Aplastic Anaemia", whereby her Bone Marrow ceases to function.

This means that Alice has severely reduced levels of red and white blood cells. Alice therefore needs regular transfusions of red cells and platelets. This condition is not common and if Alice shows no signs of improvement from her current treatment she will need a Bone Marrow Transplant.

You may not know but there is a distinct lack of Bone Marrow Donors in this country and overseas. This problem is made worse for Alice because her condition means she will need a near perfect match to prove successful.

Many friends and family have asked us about becoming a Bone Marrow Donor so we are developing this further to ask anyone who fits the criteria to take the plunge and put themselves forward as a prospective donor.

Please take time to read the leaflets before making a final decision. You may not be able to help Alice but there are many other children and adults in need of a Bone Marrow Donor.

Thank you for taking the time to read this notice please do not hesitate to contact us if you would like any further information on how to help Alice and others in need of a Donor.

WHAT CAN ___YOU___ DO TO HELP??

- If you are already a blood donor give blood as soon as possible and ask to be put on the bone marrow register. Registration takes four weeks.

- To become a new blood and bone marrow donor call the National Blood Service on 08457-711711

- If you don't want to be a blood donor but want to help call the Anthony Nolan Trust on 0901-8822234 (calls cost 25p/min and will last no longer than 3 mins). They will send you a bone marrow registration kit for you to take to your own Doctor.

For more information visit our website at: **www.helpalice.org** or email us on: **alice@helpalice.org**

Printed by Dantex Graphics Limited

08457 711 711

A printout of the home page of Alice's website: www.helpalice.org. Each time Alice's story appears in the Press it is swamped with kind messages.

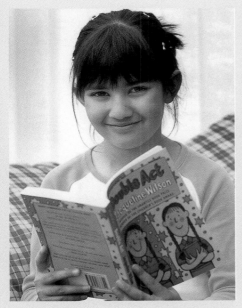

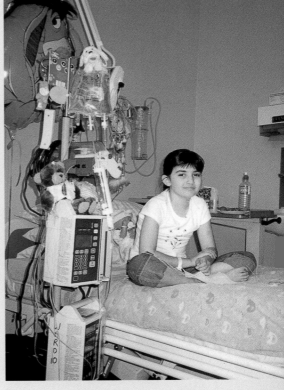

Bookworm: Alice is better than average at reading and maths despite all the school time spent in hospital.

Living in hope (right): Alice no longer minds the scores of blood transfusions needed to keep her well.

Below: Another award for the pluckiest little girl in Yorkshire.

Carol composed this prayer card (below), which was sent to thousands of Alice supporters around the world.

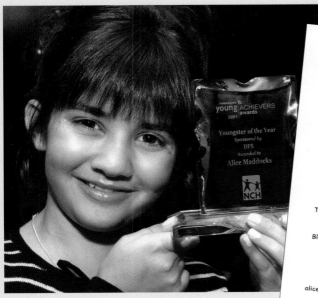

ALICE ROSE MADDOCKS
Age 8

In your prayers please remember Alice Rose as she bravely fights Aplastic-Anaemia.

Father God. Thank you for the love and care you show to Alice.

Lord keep her spirits high as she bravely fights.

Thank you Lord for the gift of Alice as she enriches our lives with her courage and love.

Bless her Lord with your healing spirit and keep her safe and free from fear.

Amen.

Email:
alice@helpalice.org

Website:
www.helpalice.org

Alice and Chloe after a spin in a West Yorkshire Police helicopter, arranged by PC Dean's fellow officers.

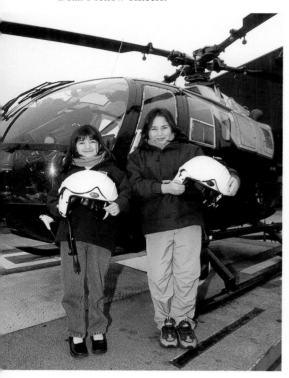

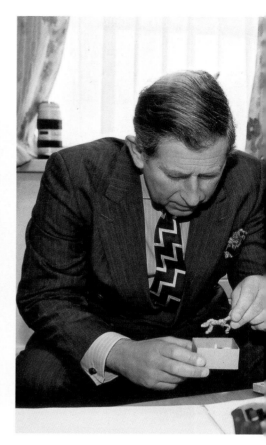

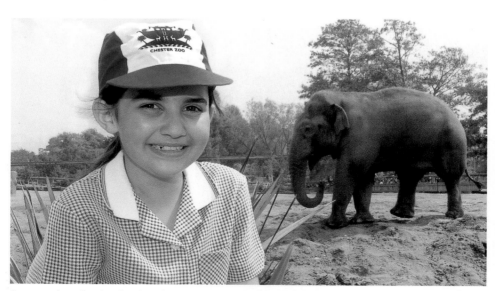

Just one day after leaving hospital treatment, pale and drawn, Alice insists on attending a long-standing treat at Chester Zoo. Dean says, 'I've never seen her so happy as that day.'

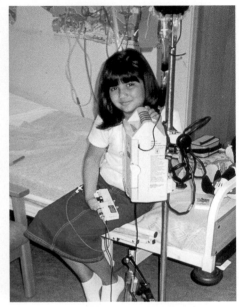

A Royal gift (left): Watched by play therapist Carol Simpson, Alice hands Prince Charles a set of 'Worry People' she made from pipe cleaners. 'He's dead posh,' she said later.

Below: Alice is never daunted by the hospital equipment needed to keep her alive.

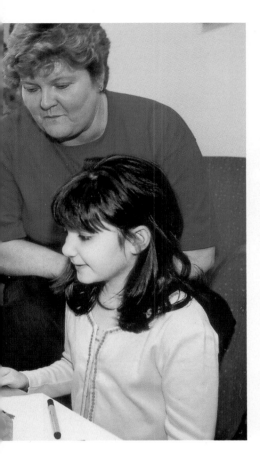

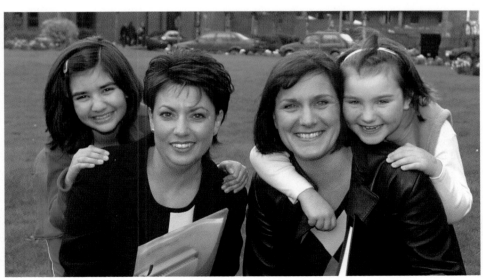

Alice and Carol with Molly-Ann Barnett and her mum Mandy – they were Carol's inspiration.

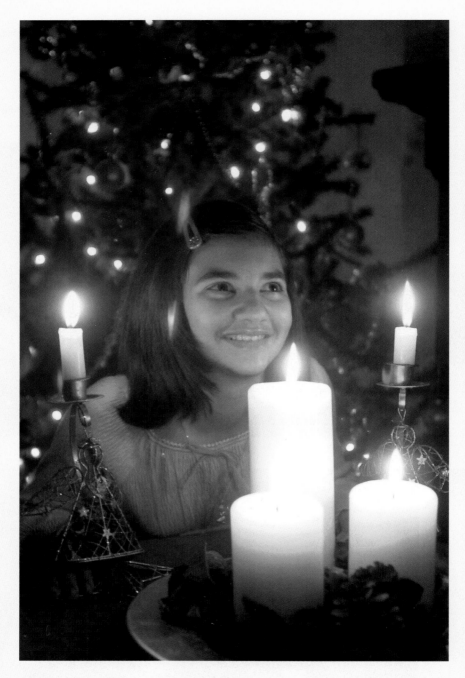

Christmas by candlelight. Alice, photographed at home for a *Yorkshire Evening Post* feature, looks back on the Maddocks' difficult year of 2002. The little girl stays cheerful throughout her ordeal.

QUESTION TIME

Please read the instructions on reverse before writing question.

Question from:-

Full name ___DEAN MADDOCKS___

Occupation ___POLICE OFFICER___

Question (maximum 30 words, in block capitals please)

THIS ELECTION IS ABOUT REAL PEOPLE WITH REAL ISSUES - SAVING OUR DAUGHTERS LIFE IS REAL TO US. MAKE A COMMITMENT NOW FOR BETTER FUNDING FOR BONE MARROW DONORS DON'T RELY ON FAMILIES AND CHARITIES FOR VITAL SERVICES

QUESTION TIME

Please read the instructions on reverse before writing question.

Question from:-

Full name ___CAROL SARA MADDOCKS___

Occupation ___Social worker.___

Question (maximum 30 words, in block capitals please)

AS PARENTS WE are alarmed TO See How Charities are funding life Saving Transplants such as The Bone marrow Registry. Our Daughter will Die Because of lack of Donors.

Two of the questions submitted by Carol and Dean to the producers of BBC TV's *Question Time*. Both were rejected.

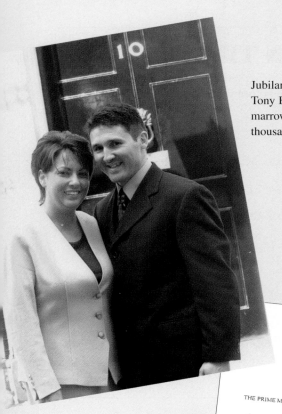

Jubilant: Carol and Dean after their get-together with Tony Blair when he promised to revitalise the bone marrow register. This one-hour meeting will save thousands of lives around the world.

Victory: Tony Blair's three-page letter to the Maddocks, in which he states that he's called for an urgent report into how to expand and invigorate the bone marrow register. It was sent via Downing Street from the Blairs' holiday hotel in Mexico.

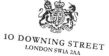

10 DOWNING STREET
LONDON SW1A 2AA

THE PRIME MINISTER

7 August 2001

Dear Dean & Carol,

    I was grateful for the chance to meet you on 24 July, and hear more about your daughter Alice and about bone marrow donor registries. Thank you, too, for your letter of 26 July

    I was very sorry to hear about Alice's illness, and the problems she faces. You explained that Alice has a very rare tissue type, and that, although efforts continue, searches of the bone marrow registries worldwide have not so far found a good match.

    As well as working to help Alice, you also want your experience to help other children in a similar position. I found our discussion on ways of improving the bone marrow registries very useful, and you explained very clearly the importance of increasing awareness and donor registration.

    We discussed the fact that the British Bone Marrow Registry achieved 17,000 new registrations last year, and the possibility of achieving 30,000 new registrations this year. This boost in bone marrow registrations is due to a considerable extent to the active campaigns, which you and others have led, to find a match for Alice and for Molly-Ann Barnett.

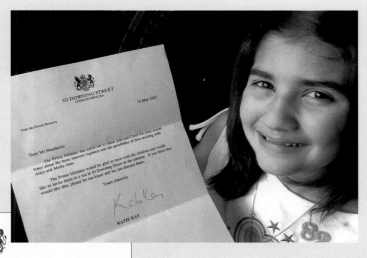

1O DOWNING STREET
LONDON SW1A 2AA

Now we need to ensure that these increases are sustained. Following our discussion I have asked the Department of Health to report to me on the following:

- What can be done to increase public awareness of the importance of becoming a bone marrow donor, and specifically informing people that they can become bone marrow donors through being a blood donor.

- How we can sustain the recent increases in bone marrow donor recruitment to achieve agreed targets for new donors of perhaps 40,000 a year, so increasing the total number of donors registered in the UK.

- What resources and funding mechanisms will best achieve this.

- How we can ensure that the three registers work together as effectively as possible.

I have asked for this report to be with me within one month. I have asked the Department of Health to keep you fully informed about the action which will be taken to improve bone marrow registration in England.

You also asked that first time blood donors be allowed to register as bone marrow donors. The National Blood Service said the reason for the current restriction was that on average only 50 per cent of new blood donors return to give blood a second time. However, you argued that this may not be the case when there is a special motivation on the part of the donor – for example, when they have responded to the needs of a particular child.

Alice is proud of her friendship with Tony Blair. This letter, inviting her to tea at Number 10, is signed by the Premier's diary secretary.

I am pleased to tell you that the National Blood Service has therefore now agreed to accept bone marrow samples from new blood donors throughout the country. This will be kept under careful review so that they can see how well it works and monitor any problems that arise.

I am glad that you were able to come and see me at such a difficult and demanding time for you and your family. Please give my best wishes to Alice. I do hope that she continues to remain well despite the rigours of her present treatment.

yours ever

Tony Blair

Children with life-threatening illnesses are entertained at No 10

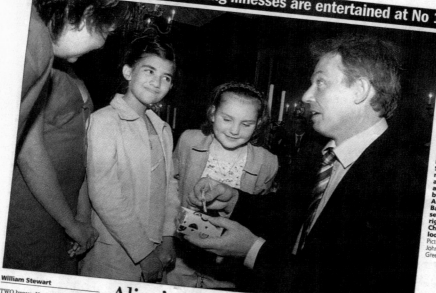

Nothing to worry about: Prime Minister Tony Blair receives worry dolls from Alice Maddocks, second left, at a Downing Street reception also attended by Molly-Ann Barnett, second right, as Cherie Blair looks on.
Picture: Johnny Green/PA

William Stewart

Alice's worry-dolls gift for Tony Blair

TWO brave Yorkshire schoolgirls took tea at 10 Downing Street yesterday in recognition of their parents' campaign to raise the number of bone marrow donors.

Nine-year-old Alice Maddocks, of Hanging Heaton, Dewsbury, who suffers from a rare life-threatening bone marrow disorder, visited the Prime Minister's home with her parents Carol and Dean.

They were joined by eight-year-old Molly-Ann Barnett, from Hull, who underwent a bone marrow transplant two years ago after succumbing to leukaemia.

The party met Cherie Blair and passed on a message of thanks to the Prime Minister for pledging an increase in donors. Mrs Maddocks said Molly had been a real inspiration to Alice, who is still waiting for a suitable donor.

Alice, who suffers from severe aplastic anaemia, said she was very excited to be at Downing Street and was feeling "very well".

Mrs Maddocks confronted Mr Blair during a special General Election edition of BBC's *Question Time* about her daughter's plight.

Following her outburst, she and her husband, a policeman, visited the Prime Minister, who pledged to raise the number of donors by an extra 40,000 a year.

Speaking as she went into No 10 Mrs Maddocks said: "We feel very positive about what they have done for us and there is now more chance that people can find a donor for Alice."

Molly-Ann, accompanied by her parents Amanda and Paul, clutched a bouquet of flowers for Mrs Blair.

Mrs Barnett said she hoped a donor would soon be found for Alice, adding: "It only takes one person.

"You stand more chance of saving Alice's life than you do of winning the lottery."

Mrs Maddocks launched a campaign [...]

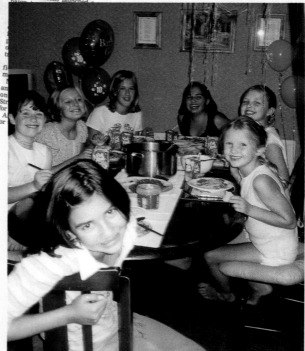

Above: The Prime Minister is 'amazed' by his gift of 'worry people', tiny figures of his family Alice made from pipe cleaners.

Alice's tenth birthday party (right) – an occasion her parents feared she would never see.

Alice and Mum at the 2002 Young Achievers Awards, a glittering dinner that was held at Leeds United's Elland Road Stadium.

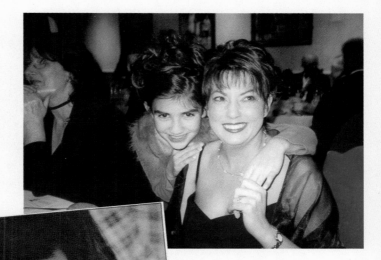

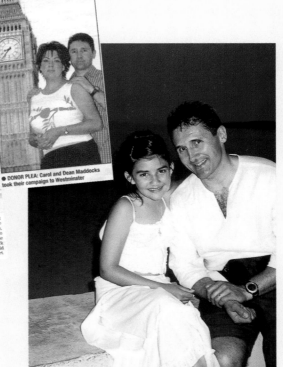

● LONG WAIT: Leukaemia sufferer Alice Maddocks. PICTURE: JAMES HARDISTY

Tony Blair's promise to help Alice find a donor by pumping millions of pounds into the bone marrow register was reported in hundreds of newspapers.

Thousands sign up for Alice donor campaign

EXCLUSIVE
BY VICKI SHAW
HEALTH REPORTER

Blair keeps his pledge – ahead of schedule

PRIME Minister Tony Blair has kept his promise to a West Yorkshire youngster – by signing up 30,000 more potential bone marrow donors.

Mr Blair pledged extra cash to boost donor numbers after an emotional meeting with the family of Dewsbury nine-year-old Alice Maddocks, who has

donor for Alice, but it's wonderful that so many other families might now get the help they need."

Dean and Carol travelled to London with Paul and Mandy

Backed by the *Yorkshire Evening Post*, they launched a campaign calling for the Bone Marrow Register to be fully funded with set targets for getting new donors.

At the meeting yesterday they were told their work had already paid off and Ministers would continue to work to boost numbers.

Dean said: "I think we got everything we could from the meeting. It was very positive, and Ms Cooper was keen to stress that she didn't see the recent emphasis as a "quick fix solution," but that it would be an ongoing concerted effort.

● DONOR PLEA: Carol and Dean Maddocks took their campaign to Westminster

A tanned Alice and Dean on holiday in Majorca, June 2002.

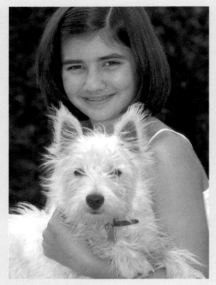

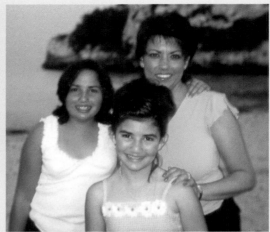

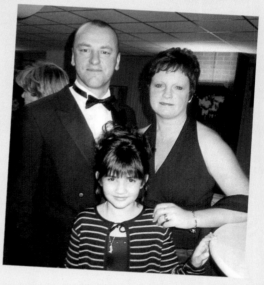

Above: Alice and her West Highland terrier, Charlie. He arrived after Mac, another terrier, who died in the early days of her illness and for whom Alice wrote a note, hoping for a reunion in heaven.

Above right: The Maddocks won't allow serious illness to spoil family fun.

Right: Sarah Walsh, Trustee of the Alice Rose Trust, and her husband, Nigel, with Alice.

Below: The Maddocks and the Barnetts, two families tirelessly campaigning for children's lives, meet Cherie Blair at Number 10.

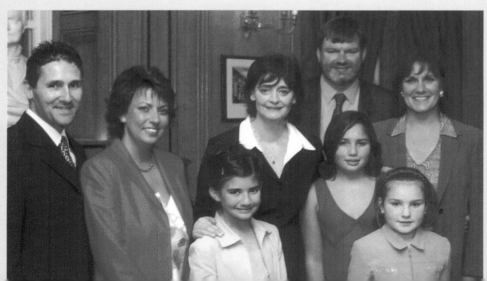

and print them out. Every organiser of every blood clinic in the North of England – and there could be as many six a day – was sent a pack of posters. These all had to be wrapped up and postage paid for. Though Dean and Carol were able to keep working during their arduous publicity mission throughout spring 2001, they still had to take Alice to St James's for regular transfusions of blood or platelets. She continued to feel sick and develop high temperatures. Each time she relapsed, it meant another five-day stay on Ward 10. In these tough circumstances Dean wondered if they could keep their fledgling campaign going much longer. Wasn't there a danger it would soon wreck their careers, squeeze their family life to death and damage the whole family's health, not just Alice's?

* * *

As they struggled with caring for Alice, their challenging jobs and their campaign, the Maddocks had a foretaste of what was to become their fourth big fish to fry in this story – a love-hate relationship with the media. It was an unholy union that would soon dominate their lives. The remarkable alliance began when a writer from their local weekly newspaper, the *Dewsbury Reporter*, noticed a 'Help Alice' poster in a café window. He was to show sensitivity to the family that was not always apparent in their future dealings with the press, television and radio. He merely pushed a note through their front door asking them to contact him, 'but only if you really want to'. Dean and Carol mulled it over for days, and then decided quite firmly... they didn't know what to do.

Dean was the charier. 'We were worried what the exposure would mean for Alice. She was sometimes so poorly she didn't even want to talk to us. Yet we knew that if we involved reporters in our lives, they would ask ticklish questions of her. They would want to photograph and film her over and over again. And we didn't want to exploit her.'

At the same time, it didn't make sense to Dean to campaign for donors and yet exclude the media from their lives. Publicity would send their message to millions, luring thousands of donors out of the woodwork. Trying to decide on the pros and cons of involving the press made their brains swim. The alternative to stirring up public interest was to sit back and wait for the National Blood Service or the Anthony Nolan Trust to find the perfect match. Their faith in that happening was getting fainter all the time. They dithered for a week, then gave a long interview to the *Dewsbury Reporter*. The can of worms was now officially open.

It's standard practice for researchers on regional TV stations to scan local papers for ideas. (Not that this filching process – known in the trade as 'lifting' – doesn't also work in reverse.) Fixers (researchers) for Yorkshire Television in Leeds were quick to spot the *Reporter* article and ask if they could interview Dean and Carol on their evening news show, *Calendar*.

Carol recoiled. 'I was petrified, absolutely frightened to death. I felt it would be like going through my driving test again. I told them I couldn't do it.' Dean, always the reticent half of the partnership, was just as nervous. But Julie Lockwood, one of *Calendar*'s most experienced news staff, persuaded the couple to co-operate. So it was that just before Christmas 2000, a van, conspicuously labelled 'Calendar', arrived at the Maddocks' home. Soon cameras were set up in the small front room, as men coiled cables and did strange things with microphones and lights.

The girls were excited, having never seen a camera crew before. But Carol and Dean were in a blue funk. Alice, however, displayed no nerves, playing to the camera with aplomb. This ability, to give TV directors exactly what they want, was to prove invaluable for the scores of TV interviews still to come, during which time Dean and Carol's nervousness faded away and Alice blossomed into a TV natural.

As they worked to secure publicity for Alice's case, Carol and Dean still sparred with local Blood Service officials who kept insisting they couldn't cope with any more volunteers. Carol felt her determination to find more donors dwindling away. 'I thought to myself I can't do any more. I don't want to do any more. I just want to curl up with Alice and for it all to go away.' But there was another force at work, tugging Carol the opposite way. Whenever she took her daughter to hospital for more tests, and found the blood count was lower, she bounced back with extra determination to find the right donor, and make Alice well. She knew the only way to boost her chances was to make Britain's bone marrow registers much bigger.

* * *

It didn't take long for the Maddocks to hit upon the idea of launching an Internet appeal for more donors. Employing a professional website designer would be too expensive. So Dean's brother-in-law Richard, a warder at Leeds Prison, recruited a friend and together they created a basic website for Alice. It wasn't an immediate success. The first two months were a wash-out. The electronic counter recorded fewer than 100 visits and most of those were from family and friends. But once Alice started to make the headlines, all that changed.

When one paper proclaimed, 'Log on to save Alice', Carol rang Richard in some excitement. 'You'll never guess what. There are 500 people on the site at the moment.' He was thrilled. But it didn't stop there. Soon the site was playing host to 1,000 visitors a day. The tally grew throughout the day: 1,200 . . . 1,500 . . . 1,750. Eventually there were more than 2,000 people wandering round the site. And they kept coming back long after that first newspaper article had been thrown away. Soon emails of support were invading the Alice's website from all over the world.

A few of the well-wishers also had aplastic anaemia. Even more had cared for family members with the disease. Some were undergoing treatment, some had recovered. Letters and emails came from Germany, France, Scandinavia, Australia, America, Europe and Mexico. They even got calls from top web designers, offering to spark up the site free of charge. One of these Samaritans was Chris Carlyle, boss of Dreamworks Webdesign, a firm based in St Helens in Lancashire. One night, after work, he drove 50 miles along the M62 between dark Satanic mills and spent many hours working with the family to produce their present sophisticated site. www.helpalice.org has not only been a lure for thousands of bone marrow donors. It has comforted the Maddocks like warm custard. Whenever they've felt let down by the professionals around them, or depressed that Alice hasn't yet found a donor, they've returned to the site's bulletin board for consolation and encouragement.

'Messages of hope come from all over the world,' said Carol, 'and that's tremendously assuring, when you consider how far behind Britain is, when it comes to finding donors.'

Occasionally the family hear about children with aplastic anaemia from other sources. One plucky little girl had been in Southampton General Hospital for many months. Her grandmother wrote to the *Daily Mail*, after hearing about Alice, telling how she's kept alive with drugs and antibiotics and how she can only be fed through a tube. A fungus had grown on her lungs making her constantly bilious with phlegm and she needed surgery to scrape it away. Only a bone marrow transplant could save her. It's stories like these that remind Carol and Dean they're not only fighting for their own daughter, but that every new name on the register could mean life for someone else.

Them and Us?

A few weeks earlier, Dean and Carol had been told by local officials in West Yorkshire that executives of the National Blood Service gathered every six weeks or so at their headquarters in London. The public wasn't excluded, but when Dean asked for details, he was informed casually, 'There's a meeting in London soon, but why not wait until the summer when they visit the north of England?' Dean, who wanted to bring his ideas right to the top of the National Blood Service, felt they couldn't afford to wait. So he made arrangements for Carol and him to go to London and lobby the meeting. Before setting off, however, they made arrangements to visit the service's labs to see at first hand how bone marrow samples were tested. The couple settled themselves down on the London train, unsure of what was to come, determined to make an impact, but quite terrified at the thought of rejection.

Staff members at the laboratories in Colindale, North London, received them warmly. They told the Maddocks of the struggles they'd had the previous year when the number of donors exceeded their capacity. They had in fact only recently cleared the backlog. They told the couple there was a need for new machines that could test several samples automatically, 24 hours a day, and which cost around £60,000 each.

Carol was impressed with their warmth and honesty and impulsively promised they would try to raise the money for those machines. Then Dean and Carol took the tube to the National Blood Service's administrative centre in the West End, brimming with optimism...

* * *

Dean thought it was like a job interview. Sitting on small chairs, the couple faced a U-shaped table surrounded by mandarins of the National Blood Service. Led by their chief executive, the urbane directors continued a good-natured debate, using lots of technical terms he and Carol couldn't understand. The pair didn't really feel welcome. They suspected these men were wondering what they were doing there at all. Hadn't they got a sick child to look after, more than 200 miles away in Yorkshire?

One of the subjects under discussion at the afternoon's meeting was a new TV campaign with former soccer star Gary Lineker. 'They seemed very pleased with that,' said Dean, 'despite the fact that the production costs would be about £100,000. I was beginning to think that money was no object.' This impression grew stronger when a financial report was read out. Apparently the service had £4 million to spend before the end of the financial year. That was little more than a month away. Carol thought that someone would suggest spending the money on the new processing machines they'd heard about earlier in the day. But instead Carol vaguely remembers a discussion on a new 'give blood' publicity campaign and a proposal to buy new vehicles.

Dean yearned to stand up and plead for a different publicity drive, aimed especially at bone marrow donors. But there was no protocol to enable him to speak at all – just to observe. Even so, the couple were happier than when they had first arrived. The National Blood Service was not short of resources as they'd feared and surely all its shortcomings were likely to be temporary.

After the formal meeting, the chief executive introduced himself. He confided that it was the first time any parents had bothered to attend one of their 'public forums'. Dean thought, 'Well at least we've made you think. You know now that at least one set of parents is watching your every move.'

Other mandarins came over to chat and the couple snatched the opportunity for some serious lobbying. Carol recalls saying to one official, 'We need more donors on the register.'

'I'm not sure we do,' he replied.

'Why?'

'Because the need is not great enough,' he pronounced.

Carol was near tears. There weren't enough donors on the register for Alice to find her match. Without that match, Alice might die. Yet this bloke was suggesting there was no need for more donors. And he was near the pinnacle of the government department running the official bone marrow register in Britain. Without complete support from the headquarters of the National Blood Service, what chance did Alice have? 'I ought to pull his head off,' she thought maliciously.

They told the chief executive of their conversation with the staff at the lab, how they needed money for new equipment to test samples. Carol became bold. 'How about earmarking some of that extra £4 million we heard you talking about?' She can't remember the chief executive's reply, only it wasn't hopeful. She can recall, however, that he seemed a bit puzzled that the couple had met some of his staff earlier. Perhaps he had not been informed.

* * *

Carol and Dean took an evening train home from King's Cross in a glum mood. The carriage was cold. They were hungry. They were so cross with the National Blood Service that they didn't even talk to each other. They'd left Leeds station with soaring hopes, sure that they could open the eyes of the National Blood Service chiefs. It may have been an ambitious aim, but they expected these civil servants to relish feedback from real live parents, anxious to improve their vital service. But now, after all that work and anticipation, they'd achieved nothing.

They'd left their seriously ill daughter for a whole day, expecting to make changes that would give her a future, but they'd failed. The National Blood Service couldn't help. They had an annual target of only 5,000 new donors a year. That was chickenfeed – and yet the executives seemed to believe they were doing all right. What could the couple do? They were on their own against an implaccable medical establishment. As their chilly railway carriage pulled into Leeds Central, the dejected pair decided to give up their crusade and concentrate on caring for Alice.

But that state of mind, born of tiredness, frustration and the lack of a buffet car, didn't last. Carol snapped awake in the early hours with the word 'No' on her lips. She spoke sternly to herself, 'We can't stop here. We'll keep our campaign going, after all. In fact, we'll build on it. We have to. We have to go all out, now. If we just wait for them, we'll never find a donor.'

Dean woke up next morning to find that his subliminal mind had made the same decision. 'We'd tried working with the National Blood Service both locally and nationally. But we realised now we would have to go it alone.'

But where should they go from here? Obviously, a drastic change of direction was called for. They decided to follow a completely new plan of action – one pioneered by Paul and Mandy Barnett. One that would ultimately save the life of their six-year-old daughter Molly-Ann ...

Molly-Ann's Story

The first I knew about Molly-Ann Barnett's fight for life was when I picked up my local weekly newspaper, the Pocklington Post

(13 July 2000). The front page headline was: 'Please Help Our Daughter' The article told how a little girl called Molly-Ann, from Hessle, a small town near the Humber Bridge, urgently needed a bone marrow transplant and urged readers to sign on as a potential donor. That's a good story, I thought, and wondered vaguely if the national press might be interested. Then I went into the garden to feed the hens. But later that day, my wife met a neighbour who sent her children to the same day nursery as our four-year-old daughter. This mother said her husband was tired out because he and everyone else at the computer software company where they worked, had undertaken a dual role. They were carrying on the normal hectic schedule of a young firm anxious to succeed and at the same time they were fund-raising for the boss's daughter, who had leukaemia. She told my wife that the money was needed to pay for special clinics to try and find a bone marrow donor for her. The girl was Molly-Ann Barnett.

With two references to the girl's plight in the same day, it seemed the story was forcing itself upon me. I reckoned that Molly-Ann could do with a helping hand from another volunteer, someone used to dealing with the press. I discovered that the case was already familiar in our neighbourhood and many local people had given their time and money. But in the rest of the country, Molly-Ann was unknown. The Pocklington Post *gave me the name and phone number of Ken Wood, marketing manager of Molly-Ann's father's software company, Viking Management Systems, which was co-ordinating the campaign. He was easily persuaded that what he and his fellow campaigners really needed was publicity for Molly-Ann's plight in the national, rather than the local press.*

I began by calling the news desks of all the national dailies, starting with those with the biggest circulation. 'I have a story which might interest you, do you want to hear it?' All the journalists sounded bored; a few suggested in desultory fashion that I send an email.

'It's about a little girl with only a week or two to live.' Bored was replaced by extremely interested and there was no more talk of emails. I gave a dramatic outline of Molly-Ann's story, together with

Ken's telephone number. All the papers put reporters on the case. Molly-Ann's parents were bombarded with phone calls, followed by visits from reporters and their photographers. Naturally, we were all looking forward to blanket coverage next day with the happy bonus of thousands of new donors. But by late afternoon I knew this wouldn't happen...

I couldn't have chosen a worse time to spread the story. I rang in my news tip on 25 July 2000, an infamous date in aviation history. As reporters filed their copy on Molly-Ann, Concorde crashed in France killing 133 people. There were dramatic films and photographs of the tragedy as it happened. Next day's newspapers ran pages and pages on this horrendous air disaster. Consequently, the story of Molly-Ann's fight for life was crowded out altogether or compressed into a paragraph or two and shunted into the back pages. Yet even the minimal coverage we had brought some response. Molly-Ann's website, artfully crafted by computer professionals free of charge, was inundated with visitors, many of whom promised to give bone marrow.

* * *

Everyone was, however, bitterly disappointed. I'd expected TV and radio stations to read the stories in the press and beat a clamorous path to Molly-Ann's door. But the path was only used by the postman the next day. What should I do now? I couldn't very well call the newspapers again with the same old tale. But there was still hope. Because television and radio news producers hadn't been able to lift the story from the papers, I could phone them with – as far as they were concerned – a new story. I waited another two days, until the Concorde story was off the boil, before ringing BBCTV News, ITN, Sky News, and the local BBC and ITV programmes. I then rang Radio 4 and Radio 5, followed by the Press Association, whose function it is to let all the media know of big news stories. Then I tried the world-wide news channels, including CNN and ABC.

This time there was no big competition from other news events, and Molly-Ann's story hit the airwaves in a satisfying way. That evening her pretty face smiled in every living room, on almost every channel in Britain. And after that, Molly-Ann's brave fight against time spread quickly around the world.

Then for me, everything went quiet. Though I was curious to know the outcome of this vast wave of publicity, I didn't make inquiries. This was because I hold a daft belief in my perverted version of an experiment in quantum physics, known as Schrödinger's Cat. The theory says, though I may have misinterpreted it, that if you leave a sick cat in a box without food, it can't be deemed to be dead – until you look at it. I take this to mean (wrongly, I expect) that if you have a problem that may or may not be solved, and you don't examine the results afterwards, everything will be all right after all. Or something like that. Though I don't really accept this theory, I didn't check up on Molly-Ann, just in case. Anyway, my mind was elsewhere. My family were just about to leave East Yorkshire to start a new life in Wales. And within a week of the big publicity drive we were much warmer in our new home in Tenby.

Three months later, our friend Janet Watson, whose husband is the Pocklington vet, came to visit us with her small son Rufus for a seaside holiday in late October at half-term. She brought the wonderful news that Molly-Ann Barnett's publicity campaign had been a success. A TV station in the United States had carried the story. As a result, two women had come forward to be tested, both of whom had exactly the right type of bone marrow. With very little time left before she would have succumbed to leukaemia, Molly-Ann was injected with healthy bone marrow cells from one of the donors. She was soon out of danger and is now living a normal life, and despite so much time in hospital, is doing very well at school.

PART TWO

A Policeman Calls

Six months later, around the middle of February 2001, one freezing Saturday morning, Dean Maddocks rang my home in Tenby. He'd heard about me from Paul and Mandy Barnett. In their usual careful way, Dean and Carol had given it a lot of thought, considered all the snags and decided to go down the same hazardous road as the Barnetts. They were intent on achieving all-out publicity. Could I help? He told me about Alice, their search for a donor and their clash with medical authorities. He was quietly spoken and reminded me of my grandfather who also came from the Dewsbury area and had the same polite telephone manner. I arranged to ring him when I'd considered the best way to launch a media campaign for his daughter.

Half an hour later, I rang Dean back and gave him a nasty shock.

'I forgot to tell you, Mr Maddocks,' I said in a my sternest Scroogesque tone, 'that I expect a rather hefty payment for undergoing this somewhat onerous work.'

There was an embarrassing silence as Dean's stomach tightened. Paul hadn't warned him about this. This Malcolm might, at best, be a greedy so-and-so; at worst a con man.

'I'm afraid we didn't expect a fee ... you see, we ...'

'My going rate is ...' (I paused cruelly to build the suspense) 'that Alice has to send me a letter telling me how she spent her eighteenth birthday. Because I can see into the future – and she will be having one.'

Another silence ...

'Well, do I get my fee or shall we forget all about it now?'

'I think it can be arranged,' said a much happier Dean.

Afterwards I felt a pang of remorse. This was not the sort of joke to play on a father in Dean's position. But money hadn't been discussed during the first phone call, and I'd wanted an easy way of telling him none was expected.

(I did not like to admit to Dean that I had never given blood. I just can't do it. The prospect of volunteering bone marrow would, I'm sure, present a similar reaction. Cravenly I was guiltily rather relieved that I'm just over the age limit of 45.)

Raring as I was to start our media offensive as quickly as possible, I had to warn Dean that there might not be a repetition of the rush of reporters to the Barnetts' door. The stories of both girls were very similar. News editors might not yet be ready to go down the same route. They generally obey the law of diminishing returns and avoid 'compassion fatigue'. A certain amount of craftiness was called for if we wanted to make a splash. I'd kept a list of all the health correspondents who'd taken an interest in Molly-Ann, but I decided not to contact them again. They would undoubtedly remember the previous story, and might be bored by another bone marrow search. Instead I asked to speak to a general reporter.

The approach was the same as last time, 'Can I offer you a cracking good story?' Again the response of polite – and sometimes not so polite – disinterest. You can understand it. Journalists are forever getting calls from people wearing bonnets with bees in them, flogging tired issues and non-stories, which they believe to be fascinating. Only one in 30 calls from the public ever leads to anything. On the other hand, journalists are keen to tackle tales that don't originate in press hand-outs or foreseen events in the news diary. So nobody tried to brush me off. And it would be hard indeed to resist my next line, 'It's about an eight-year-old child with very little time to live.' That did it! The reporters were very attentive now. And if any had remembered the Molly-Ann case, they didn't mention it.

I had worked with Dean on an emotive, tear-jerking press release. We either faxed or emailed it to reporters as soon as they replaced the receiver after my initial call. The hand-out was a bare outline of Alice's fight, just enough to spark interest. It had the Maddocks' home number, separate mobile numbers for Dean and Carol and their address. I also stressed that the family would help journalists in every way possible. This would please the hacks who rarely get full co-operation, even from people who woo their attention.

Some reporters asked if they could have the story on an exclusive basis. It was a forlorn hope: Alice obviously needs the widest coverage possible. One optimistic man asked if I would delay letting others papers know, as he was busy doing something else. I regretfully declined and added, 'The trouble is that everybody else is already besieging Alice's front door.' It was an old trick, but I knew the fear of competition would spur him on.

* * *

Having worked my way through the national newspapers, I wondered if I should call a halt. If the story had half decent headlines tomorrow, television and radio stations would follow it up, anyway. If the newspapers didn't go with Alice's story, then I could – as in Molly-Ann's case – ring up the broadcasters and try to persuade them to carry it later. It was a difficult decision. In the end, as little news seemed to be breaking, I thought why not, so I dialled BBC television and radio news, ITN, GMTV and Sky News.

Normally if someone calls in with a tip-off, the BBC circulates all its news and current affairs programmes. But this was no time to take chances. I also rang producers working exclusively for BBCTV *Breakfast News* and the *Six O'Clock News*. Then I left a message for the BBC's health correspondent Neil Dixon. Finally I went back to my favourite pastime – staring gormlessly at the sea.

But at the Maddocks' home, all hell had broken loose.

Unleashing the Beast

The eager dash by journalists to gather words and pictures about Alice was even more enthusiastic than the rush to grab the Molly-Ann Barnett story. All our national papers carried 'Alice' articles and pictures. So did a cluster of TV news and radio programmes. Many people strive for years to win publicity at this level – and still fail. The Maddocks family, co-operative, photogenic and full of sublime quotes, had a stunning success at their first try. As a result of this first sortie into the world of national news, tens of thousands of well-wishers logged on to www.helpalice.org and in surgeries up and down the land people asked their doctors how to give bone marrow.

The couple had high hopes that at least one of these new donors would prove to be Alice's saviour. After all, she'd already had nearly as much exposure as Molly-Ann, who'd found her donor and was now safe. But no one would be sure for some months. So Dean and Carol, already over-stretched by their jobs and looking after Alice, vowed to keep the publicity pot boiling, by thinking up new 'angles' whenever they could. When they found them – and there's always a dramatic development in Alice's story – they telephoned me in Tenby and I told the press immediately.

This was the couple's first encounter with the British media at a national level. And in many ways, they were pleasantly surprised. For example, they found reporters were courteous and sympathetic. They seemed genuinely concerned about Alice. The kindly approach is, of course, a main tool of the trade. You don't get stories by being brusque and unfeeling. In fact, the more adept the reporter, the better his or her bedside manner.

But the Maddocks still had some disturbing questions to deal with, some of which showed a few journalists in a less considerate light. One or two unfeeling hacks blandly pressed the couple on how long Alice could be expected to live. Researchers from one TV programme even suggested they couldn't possibly carry the story unless they knew this fact. Dean was the most indignant about this line of questioning. 'Can you imagine how damaging that would have been to Alice; to overhear us saying she would die in a few weeks without a bone marrow transplant? Did they really expect us to do that? That wasn't our message at all – we just wanted to appeal for more donors and the extra cash to process them.'

* * *

An unspoken quid pro quo stalks the media jungle. Reporters who're given sensation and controversy will show their gratitude by adding the more prosaic details if requested. So I advised Dean and Carol to do deals. They should make the story of Alice dramatic and heart-warming, without resorting to lies. In return they could reasonably demand that the newspaper publish a direct appeal for donors, ideally with clear instructions on how to sign up, together with the address of Alice's website. Dean and Carol took to media manipulation like ducks to water. Indeed, they were soon teaching me how to tame the wolf pack.

Two Goals for Sister Sarah

When she first realised how seriously ill Alice was, Carol's first instinct was to turn to Sarah Walsh who'd been her best friend for fourteen years. But when she rang her home, Sarah's husband Nigel said she was abroad on holiday. At first Carol couldn't wait for her confidante, whom she regarded as a sister, to return home. But then her impatience to see Sarah jerked to a halt. Carol developed a superstitious dread that once she told her friend that a mystery illness threatened Alice, the final diagnosis would be devastating. But she was spared from telling her as Nigel phoned his wife in Greece to explain what was happening to Alice. The first thing Sarah did on coming home was to phone Carol to offer support. Since then, the two friends have seen each other every day to discuss Alice – and spoken by phone many more times than that.

Despite being a full-time social worker, Sarah became a second mother to Chloe, while Dean and Carol devoted so much time to Alice in hospital. She opened her home to the older girl, treating her in bowling alleys, shopping malls, the cinema and the seaside. Her own daughters, twenty-year-old Laura and seventeen-year-old Abi, became Chloe's older sisters. All this care and attention for Chloe was extremely welcome to Dean and Carol, who constantly worried that their elder daughter would feel left out. But they still felt uneasy about putting on Sarah, even if she's happiest doing favours for friends. 'She's that strange kind of person who would burn herself out for the sake of others,' said Carol.

Sarah set herself twin goals for Alice – to make her well and happy again and to ease the weight on her parents' shoulders. To help her achieve both aims, Sarah suggested setting up a trust fund for Alice. The idea came to her during her first visit to see the little girl in hospital. But when she first mentioned it, she was flabbergasted to find her friend was horrified by the idea. Carol explained that the only trusts of that kind she'd heard about were for children who were desperately unwell and could die. She wasn't ready to put Alice in that drab pigeonhole. She also proudly believed the family would never need extra money to care for Alice. No, a trust for Alice Maddocks was definitely out of court!

* * *

Sarah, however, had other ideas. And she hatched her plans under cover of a girls' weekend in Blackpool.

Every August for the previous thirteen years, Sarah had arranged a 'fun weekend' for herself, Carol and a gang of old friends. Originally, they were keen to sample the neon lights of discos and rowdy nightclubs. But the object of their annual trip changed as the group matured. They still wore their smart evening outfits, but began to spend more of their time indoors, chatting and catching up on recent events. These were real 'girly times' spent among trusted friends. This friendship had grown over many years and was now an integral part of their lives, a real institution.

As Alice recovered from her first round of hospital treatment, the fourteenth annual Blackpool jaunt was imminent. Carol decided Alice needed her at home, but her friends had other ideas. Dean and the two girls also felt she deserved the break. So Carol packed, only to change her mind just before the departure. She put her bags down in the hall and refused to move. But Dean wasn't having it, and with some small loss to her dignity, physically shoved her out of the front door.

So Carol, Sarah, Angela, Karen, Julie, Denise, Diane and Sarah's daughter, Laura, descended on their homely rented apartment near Blackpool's Golden Mile. They planned to spend most of the weekend in the lounge, just having an elongated natter. Helping pass the time were bottles of wine and boxes of chocolates – and an unwritten rule that they share each other's perfumes, face-creams and bubble bath stuff. In between joking and gossiping, clowning about and telling old jokes, the main subject for debate at the big get-together was Alice's illness. It was the first time most of the group had had a chance to hear what had happened at first hand. They tried hard to make Carol think there was nothing to worry about. And for two happy days the constant worry of Alice's health faded. Meantime, a discussion was going on behind her back. The other women all agreed, whether she liked it or not, that they would set up the 'Alice Rose Trust'.

Carol knew nothing about this pact, until her return home. Then Sarah announced that everybody in the group was giving money to start a bank account especially for Alice. She braced herself for an angry refusal. But though there was still need for some persuasion, it wasn't as much as Sarah expected. By this time Carol, always the pragmatist, was beginning to see that money could indeed run short if she and Dean continued to neglect their jobs to care for Alice. Even so, both still nursed some reluctance towards starting a trust fund. They wouldn't voice any plausible reason against it, but secretly they were just too proud to live on charity.

The couple looked for more practical reasons to stifle the idea. Surely, they told Sarah, there would be complicated legal hoops to go through. Costly accountants would have to be involved. And wouldn't they need to approach the Charity Commission for a licence? 'No need to worry,' said Sarah reassuringly. It was all surprisingly simple to set up a trust fund. She'd made inquiries, and found they could easily arrange a dedicated bank account. All that was needed were specimen signatures from two of the group who would act as trustees.

Still the couple were not sure. But Sarah never gives up easily – if at all. She applied more coercion on Carol and Dean. 'What if you can't pay your phone bill? What are you going to do if you can't put petrol in your car? And what will happen if Alice needs a holiday?' Finally, Dean and Carol gratefully caved in – and the Alice Rose Trust was born. (Alice's middle name was added to the Trust for the same reason it was added to the website, because it rolls easily off the tongue.)

* * *

The 'friends of Alice Rose' didn't allow their money to fester in the bank for long. They'd heard Carol describe how Alice was frightened of her own bedroom after returning from hospital. So they insisted that the Trust's first cash grant should transform the room to Alice's taste. That would dispel her fear all right! A cheque was drawn for paint, wallpaper, curtains and wood to make new furniture. Dean wasn't truly happy with this arrangement. He was troubled over using somebody else's money to redecorate his own home. So Sarah brokered a compromise.

Though he agreed that the Trust could pay for materials, he refused to allow any tradesman over the threshold. He did all the work himself – the painting, wallpapering and even the carpentry. Yet his time was very limited, because of the demands of his police duties and his regular hospital visits. Thus hampered, it took Dean two months to paint the bedroom in lilac and pale yellow, and saw, plane, hammer and screw together a suite of snazzy cupboards and shelves. The room was equipped with a new combined television and video recorder. Colleagues in the West Yorkshire police had a whip-round for that. And there was a collection of small toy bears, sent by one of Carol's workmates. It was all worth it in the end. Instead of Alice fearing to enter her room, it was now difficult to keep her out of it!

While the bedroom was transformed, money started to pour into the Trust, thanks to an epidemic of fund-raising events in Dewsbury area. This stream of revenue would have pleased most parents with a child in constant need of medical attention. They would have regarded a steady supply of cash from a trust, run by golden-hearted volunteers, as well-deserved. And why not? When you're struggling through a tough patch, money greases the chute, makes a difficult

life and harrowing prospects easier to cope with. But Dean and
Carol are not run-of-the-mill parents. The founding of Alice's fund
was a flea, nibbling at their conscience. They couldn't accept charity
just to improve their lives – not unless it was unavoidable. And so
far, though Carol's income in particular was heavily eroded by the
growing burden of caring for Alice, they were coping.

Eventually, as always happens with thoughtful people, their
consciences won out. They decided to ask the 'friends of Alice
Rose' if they could arrange for the Trust to support other families as
well as their own. They also suggested some money be used to buy
equipment for the children's wards at St James's Hospital. Both felt
much happier with this new arrangement. The 'friends of Alice
Rose', however, were not about to let what they regarded as
misplaced sensitivity dictate to them in every respect. They insisted
that the Trust should supply the Maddocks' home with a computer,
fax machine, two mobile phones, a micro cassette recorder, stacks
of envelopes and reams of typing paper. All this would be needed to
keep the campaign for donors running in top gear.

Then the Trust bought the family a camcorder to tape any happy
times they might still have left. Said Carol, 'Though we pushed it to
the back of our minds, we were all aware Alice might not be with us
for long. So we were grateful for that camcorder. We used it a lot,
just to preserve the good moments.' The Trust also paid a
photographer to produce a set of family portraits, because at the
time it seemed Alice might lose her long hair.

* * *

The 'friends of Alice Rose' finally agreed to Dean and Carol's wish
to include other charities and individuals on the Trust's benefit list.
They could afford to. Alice's plight had touched a chord in West
Yorkshire and the money was rolling in. The Trust was soon able to
support big charities, like the Anthony Nolan Trust and local
hospitals, including St James's and the Dewsbury District. But
naturally enough, Dean and Carol were happiest helping individual
children. At one fund-raising event for the Trust, a small blind boy,
with the voice of an angel, sang 'My Heart Will Go On' for Alice.
Carol discovered later that his parents were saving up for a braille

computer. The 'friends of Alice Rose' shelled out £500 – half the proceeds from the evening – to buy it. Money also came from Alice's trust for a little girl who spent ten hours daily on a kidney dialysis machine and for a ten-year-old cancer patient whose ambition is to swim with dolphins.

Esther

Occasionally I made appearances on the *Esther* show on BBC2. My subject was money, something dear to my heart. While chatting in the bar after one recording, I mentioned Alice's crusade to one of the production team. Though I expected him to be as interested as a vegetarian in roast beef, I left the Maddocks' telephone number on the slight chance Alice's story might be included in a future programme. On a Saturday evening about two weeks afterwards, the Maddocks' phone rang. Carol was amazed to hear a very familiar voice. Esther wasn't calling to book the Maddocks for a programme on child health. She just wanted to know how Alice was.

Carol didn't need to explain all the medical technicalities of severe aplastic anaemia. Esther already knew about the illness, rare though it is. She spent nearly half an hour talking to Alice's mum, encouraging her in the fight to find a donor and making suggestions to further the campaign.

Later, Esther sent a letter to Alice from her home in North London. 'I think of you a great deal – I do hope you're feeling a lot better. With loads of love, Esther'. Alice sent Esther a reply. Out of the envelope fell a set of 'worry people', including a star, fashioned from pipe cleaners. With it came a message in Alice's neat handwriting, 'This is for Desmond who is now a star in Heaven.' Esther's husband, the documentary film maker Desmond Wilcox had died about a year before. Esther was touched. She said later,

'That little girl is so ill, yet she found the strength to send me something as wonderful as that.'

Esther Rantzen swung behind the Maddocks' campaign to make it easier for blood donors to put their name down to give bone marrow. She went on the record with, 'There are so many blood donors in this country. It would so easy for them when they fill in their forms to tick a box saying they're happy to be included on the bone marrow register as well,' adding, 'I can't understand why the authorities don't do it.'

Carol learned later that Esther has a personal interest in organ donations. Desmond Wilcox had given his name as an organ donor. After he was struck down by a heart attack, doctors were able to transplant his bones, skin and tissue into people who would have died otherwise.

There was a twist to the story of Esther's kind interest in Alice. The television star later asked for Alice to be featured several times on her Sunday morning ITV series, *That's Esther*. This programme was inadvertently to cause a big headache for the Maddocks' publicity drive, but more on that later...

Sir Alex

Alice's fame soon spread everywhere, not least on the Internet. Many kind people were putting www.helpalice.org on their own websites, large and small, business and private. This is the big advantage of the net. There's an all-for-one mentality out there whereby people who're complete strangers help each other. I lodged Alice's web address and an appeal for bone marrow onto Sharecrazy.com, a forum for private investors in stocks and shares. Consequently, hundreds of goodwill messages flowed onto the site's message board.

A business contact told Alice's story to Alex Ferguson, manager of Manchester United. Both were unaware that Alice is a keen United fan but Sir Alex decided to help anyway.

Within a few days of his hearing about Alice, two huge parcels arrived at the Maddocks' home. Inside were United T-shirts, scarves, badges and a gigantic teddy bear. With this wonderful hoard came a club membership card with Alice's name on it. There was a letter from Sir Alex, too.

Dear Alice,

I'm sorry to hear of your health problems.

I just thought I would drop you a wee line, as I wanted you to know that the players and myself are thinking about you.

I know that the last few months have been difficult for you, but trust that you will gain some comfort knowing that you are in our thoughts and prayers.

God bless

Sir Alex Ferguson CBE
MANAGER

For Alice this was a lovely surprise. Her bedroom walls were already covered with posters of Manchester United stars and for as long as Dean could remember it had been hs favourite team, too. As ecstatic as Alice, he phoned the club to give his thanks and was promptly invited to take Alice across the Pennines to meet the team. The pair watched the team beat Coventry City with four blistering goals. It was Alice's first football match, and although unwell, she thrilled to each minute. Afterwards they were taken to the players' bar to meet the victors. All her heroes were there – Andy Cole, Nicky Butt, Roy Keane, Ryan Giggs and Teddy Sheringham. They made a huge fuss of the little girl and wished her well. That night Dean told Carol that if Alice's life was to be curtailed by aplastic anaemia, then at least she was making the most of it.

S Club 7

Though her parents try hard not to spoil Alice, they do feel that if her life is to be short, then it should be enriched with as many excitements as possible. So they shelled out for tickets to an S Club 7 pop concert at the Sheffield Arena, about 40 minutes' drive away. Maybe we can do better than that, I thought. Perhaps the teenage group might agree to meet Alice backstage if they knew her story. I phoned the management at the Arena, and asked them to pass on the request. They agreed to approach the tour organisers.

'Alice is going to be cock-a-hoop,' I reflected. 'It's about time she had some fun.' But it began to look as though the meeting with S Club 7 wouldn't happen after all. With Saturday almost upon us, I'd still heard nothing. Neither had the Sheffield Arena. I rang the BBC. The corporation has a department called 'Artist's Index', which puts producers in touch with performers and actors. But even they couldn't trace a phone number for the agents. Now time really was slipping by. Our inquiries needed to widen and fast.

I tried the Internet, looking for show biz agents who would possibly handle famous groups. I found one and asked if they represented S Club 7. No, but they knew a man who did. Normally, you might expect workers in the rough tough pop world to be uncooperative. But then I wasn't sensitive about telling Alice's tale with all the emotive stops pulled out. I left an urgent message with the agent's office for someone with authority on the tour to contact me. I rather doubted anybody would, given the hectic nature of pop group tours, but I left a description of the Maddocks family, in case some kind person connected with S Club 7 might recognise them in the Arena and arrange something. But nothing happened. Alice saw the show, loved it, but sadly did not meet her idols backstage. Wisely, Dean and Carol never mentioned to her that this was a possibility.

But we are a kindly nation and later the Maddocks had a letter from S Club 7. 'We send our love to Alice and our thoughts are with her family and friends.' And they added, 'We wish the Maddocks luck with their campaign and encourage all blood donors to join the bone marrow register.' The family never discovered if any of the group joined the register themselves, but Alice did meet her idols when they returned to Sheffield a few months later.

An older pop star who has contacted the family to offer support is Brian May, from Queen. He wrote to say: 'The more people who volunteer for possible donation of a tiny piece of the bone marrow material some time in the future – the more chance we have of saving not only Alice, but thousands of children in the years to come.' And many more famous people have written to Dean and Carol offering encouragement and hope – including Esther Rantzen.

The Prince and the Worry People

On 9 February 2001 Alice went to St James's Hospital to meet a very dapper, middle-aged man who arrived in a chauffeur-driven Bentley. The Prince of Wales was there to formally open the Robert Ogden Centre, built in the grounds for the recreation of cancer patients and partly financed by the hospital and the Macmillan Cancer Relief charity. Alice was specially chosen to meet the Prince there.

But the first six children he came across in the hospital refused to speak to him. Instead, they held up a placard: 'Sorry we can't talk to you. We are doing a sponsored silence. It's to raise money for people with cancer.'

Soon afterwards, the Prince, wearing a red carnation, walked into the centre where Alice was waiting for him in a private room. The little girl looked up, smiled and shyly handed His Royal Highness a small, decorated, trinket box.

'What's this?' he asked.

'It's a worry box.'

The Prince carefully opened the lid. The box contained a few figures she'd made from coloured pipe cleaners similar to the ones she had given to Esther Rantzen. They were in the form of Princes William and Harry, the Queen Mother and a horse.

'These are worry people,' she told him gleefully. 'They live in the box.'

'And what should I do with them?'

'You can tell the worry people about your problems and they listen. And when you shut the box, your worries get smaller.' She paused, her face a little more serious. 'I thought it would be nice if you had some worry people to talk to.'

'Thank you, they'll be most useful,' said the Prince. And he gave her a warm smile. Alice spent the next quarter of an hour chatting casually with her new friend, the future King of England, while Mum, Dad and Chloe stood nervously outside. The Prince left Alice and walked over to Dean and Carol. 'How do you cope with something so dreadful?' he asked compassionately. They answered by speaking about their great hope of finding a matched bone marrow donor. He went on to tell them how fortunate he was that his children had not suffered any serious illness. He marvelled at the Maddocks' positive attitude to the situation. Then they all swapped jokes with other guests, Liz Dawn, who plays Vera Duckworth in *Coronation Street*, and the Lady Mayoress of Leeds.

Little did the Prince know about the family conversations leading up to this big day. Alice had been concerned about how many worry people she should make for him. 'Shall we make one of Princess Diana?' she asked, and after much debate decided against it, but as children often do, Alice went on to present her parents with a much more awkward question, 'What about Camilla?'

Asked afterwards what she thought of Prince Charles, Alice said, 'He was very nice – and very posh.'

Help and Hindrance

Like it or not, the Maddocks family has become known as the 'Fastidious Campaigners' of West Yorkshire. Everybody has read about their sad tale in the papers or seen them on television. It seems the entire population feels sorry for Alice, sympathises with Chloe and admires their beleaguered parents. Everybody wants to help, too. Think of the 'Children in Need' epic on BBC TV every autumn. Something very similar happens in Yorkshire all the time – but there's only one beneficiary – the Alice Rose Trust. Few of those who raise cash for the cause realise that only a fraction goes to help the family. But then Yorkshire folk don't always care what happens to the money as long as they have the pleasure of raising it. True, the same people can sometimes be a bit hesitant to dip in their own pockets, but they love staging events to prise money from their fellow citizens.

The fund-raising carnival began in a small way. Elderly residents of Manorcroft Nursing Home in Dewsbury started the ball rolling with a raffle. One of the staff then persuaded her husband to run a couple of discos at the Old Anchor pub down the road. News of the recently formed Alice Rose Trust then spread through newspaper coverage of those first two events.

Neighbours took £500 at a coffee morning in the Methodist Church. Local singer Ricky Alan performed free at Hanging Heaton Working Men's Club. England rugby league star, Darren Fleary, signed a rugby ball and shirt, and so did his team mates from the 2000 World Cup squad. The *Yorkshire Evening Post* auctioned the shirt for £250 and the ball for £300. A smart clothes shop in nearby Mirfield organised a fashion show in the Mandarin Chinese restaurant, using firemen as unlikely models. Some 200 tickets were sold and the event raised £3,000. As time went on, the Trust's sources of money became even more prestigious. At a social highlight of the year, the Mayor of Kirklees Annual Dinner in Huddersfield, £1,400 was raised for the Trust.

Dean and Carol went to most of these functions and were very grateful for them. But they didn't enjoy every moment. From the time they walked through the door to the minute they left, a cavalcade of kind-hearted people would ply them with questions about Alice. The Maddocks, appreciative of anyone who was concerned for Alice, reluctantly found themselves talking about her in intimate detail – from her chances of survival to how she managed in the toilet!

'People always think we're having a good night out,' said Dean, 'but really we can't relax for a minute. We have to keep telling the same old stories, over and over again. It's exhausting, but we feel we have to keep up our sickly smiles for Alice's sake.'

When they feel they just can't face another event, the couple sometimes beg members of the 'friends of Alice Rose' to go in their place. But this doesn't always go down well. 'They want us there in person,' Carol lamented. 'They need us to act the part of local celebrities. But we never see ourselves like that. We're a normal family who've been forced by cruel fate into this media jungle. We have no choice but to go down the publicity route. People can't understand that. They can't separate us from people who're happy to be in the limelight because they're sports or show biz personalities. Everyone seems to think our appearances in public are something we revel in.'

* * *

This view of Alice as a child star, a sort of Shirley Temple, pervades all aspects of life in West Yorkshire. One dreary December morning, a stranger stopped Carol in the street and asked if Alice could read a poem in Dewsbury Minster. The woman obviously expected her to be flattered and delighted to say 'yes'. But instead Carol was appalled. She asked herself, 'Why can't people think? My little girl is very young, very ill and fighting for life itself. And yet this person expects her to stand up alone in front of hundreds of people and read to them. Is she mad?' Carol didn't put her angry thoughts into words, but she was still quite curt with the woman. 'I'm sorry but I can't think of anything worse for Alice to do. She would be mortified.' And she walked away, rather abruptly.

Dean supports his wife in refusing to put Alice on a pedestal. 'These people don't know Alice from Adam. They don't know us, either. They've just seen us in the papers. Their hearts are in the right place, but maybe not their heads.'

The strain sometimes led the couple to consider abandoning the Alice Rose Trust Fund to concentrate on Alice's hospital visits and their campaign to drum up more donors. But when they think how much Trust money has already helped sick children and cash-strapped hospitals, they soon relent. More pragmatically, they admit they can't keep their campaign going unless the Trust continues to pay most of the expenses. So the Alice Rose Trust is secure and thriving, and as a result thousands of seriously ill children are much better off.

Just thinking about the benefits of the Trust gives Dean and Carol a lot of comfort in their tortured lives. But while the pair is very grateful to their many genuine supporters, they've discovered something out there in the fund-raising world that has utterly shocked them. There are people willing to exploit Alice for their own shady ends...

* * *

Some events have been staged in the little girl's name, raising cash that was never given to the Alice Rose Trust. It just disappeared into somebody's pocket. Less dishonest, but just as annoying, are people who arrange events in Alice's name for hidden motives. Organisers have either creamed off a hefty slice of commission, or they've made a mint out of people buying drinks, once inside the pub or similar venue. Sometimes they've staged an Alice Rose event only to snare publicity for their own business.

Then there are the local firms who offer to mount some kind of fund-raising shindig – but only if the Maddocks can guarantee television or newspaper coverage. 'They know we have a media following, and they're more concerned with milking that than raising money to help Alice and other sick kids,' said Dean. The couple used to fall for it at first, 'But we soon learned to have nothing to do with people like that.'

They admit they've taken quite a few false trails as they wander round the publicity maze. But then nothing in the Maddocks' life ever runs smoothly. For example, on one occasion a well-intentioned public relations company asked Alice to switch on the Christmas lights at a large shopping centre in Batley on 15 November 2001. Naturally enough, the little girl jumped at the idea – at first.

There's a toy shop in the complex and the firm suggested that Alice should pick out some of the stock to give to the Robert Ogden Centre, the new children's day facility in the grounds of St James's Hospital. When they arrived at the shopping centre, Dean and Carol were surprised to find that Alice wasn't the only child chosen to pick toys. The organisers had also invited a group of children from a local rugby club. These kids rushed at the shelves in a frenzy of excitement. While it was nice to see them having such fun, they picked out many toys that were unsuitable, mainly because they wouldn't last two minutes in the day centre. Alice wasn't at all happy with the final choice. Helpers at the day hospital had told her what they wanted her to choose – strong, robust playthings – like Lego or Brio sets. The pile of toys before her contained nothing like that. But still, it couldn't be helped and the toy shop had certainly been generous. So Dean and Carol comforted their daughter and prepared her for the next stage of the event.

Alice pushed down a giant plunger in an electrical box and turned on the Christmas lights surrounded by TV cameras, press photographers and reporters. It sounds like a huge honour, something which only big celebrities ever do. But the family soon wished they weren't there. This was nothing to do with the event, which was well-staged and popular with the crowd, but the sad fact that Alice was unwell again. After a transfusion earlier in the day, she now felt sick and had a headache. Even so, a game Alice smiled earnestly and did everything the photographers wanted her to.

After the switch-on ceremony, Dean offered to take all the chosen toys to St James's the next time they had an appointment. But the organisers had other plans. They wanted to surprise the young patients at St James's by bringing Santa along to hand over the goodies. Would Alice like to join him? Of course she would. However, when the Maddocks arrived at the day centre, they found a boisterous reception committee – all their usual friends from the local television stations and newspapers.

An annoyed 'Dr Mike' quickly bearded Alice's parents. He was upset by the media circus in his hospital and thought they'd orchestrated the affair for yet more coverage. Dean and Carol were mortified that anyone could believe they would deliberately generate a publicity stunt in the midst of sick children. It must have seemed to 'Dr Mike' that the couple would do anything just to get their faces on television. Some chilly words were exchanged between the nurses and the firm organising the event. In the end, the hospital allowed limited photo coverage of Santa's handing-over ceremony at the Robert Ogden Centre.

When Santa asked Alice what she wanted him to bring in his sack, he was a little bemused by her answer, 'All I want for Christmas is a high platelet count.'

During St Nick's visit to the centre, Alice bravely undertook two hours of press photography and filming. Carol Simpson, one of the play centre staff, was watching her closely. As photographers pleaded for 'just a few more shots', she stepped in and retorted 'Enough is enough!' She recognised that Alice was jaded and tired and didn't want to do this anymore. Dean backed her up, calling an immediate halt to the affair. He was learning that sometimes journalists expect too much, and after the Christmas lights affair, he vowed never to allow publicity stunts to upset Alice again.

* * *

Meanwhile the Alice Rose Trust kept on growing as fund-raising events continued unabated. Alice's 34-year-old Uncle Tony went on a sponsored bike trip from Land's End to John O'Groats. 'The family have such a lot on, I just wanted to show my support,' he said. Three policemen from Dean's division showed the force was with Alice by running thirteen sponsored miles from Newcastle-upon-Tyne to South Shields.

Sometimes money was given to the Trust from unexpected sources. Like the time the Whirly Birds Appeal, a unique charity set up by Dewsbury bus drivers, ceased to exist. Twice a year, they used to take 100 kids from nearby hospitals to Blackpool for trips in helicopters and wild rides on the beach in fast cars. Sadly, the founder David Crowther had to stop organising this exciting venture to care for his wife Julie who'd developed multiple sclerosis. The charity was wound up and its remaining £1,800 was given to Alice's Trust. Dean and Carol accepted the cash – and bought a much-needed piece of equipment for Dewsbury District Hospital. This was the comically named pulsoximeter, a device for measuring pulse rates and the volume of oxygen in a patient's blood.

With money from the Alice Rose Trust, Dean and Carol began to organise their own clinics to take samples from people who wanted to become donors. These sessions cost about £5,000 each. It may seem a lot of money, but it's a complex, costly business to take and store blood. Expensive hi-tech equipment is needed. Some of these temporary clinics had unlikely venues. One was at Dewsbury's rugby league stadium, home of the 'Rams'. One wet Saturday afternoon, Alice was the Rams' mascot for their match with Widnes Vikings. She ran onto the field with the team, almost hidden behind the club's orange, yellow and black scarf. Next day, she was guest of honour at the seven-hour session itself. Nearly 300 of the club's fans turned up to give samples. These were processed, on their day off, by staff from the district hospital.

Alice's school friends twice persuaded their teachers to hold blood donor sessions in the school. About 170 volunteers attended each session. All donors were specifically asked if they would also agree to join the bone marrow register, and most did.

The business world has also been moved by Alice's story. One company printed 5,000 posters with Alice's face and an appeal for bone marrow. The owners of a firm called Fresco read about the appeal in the papers, and donated a huge electronic notice board. The Maddocks regard this clever apparatus as 'a godsend'. They take it with them to all their clinics and cash-raising events. It flashes up all the news on Alice, how to become a donor and a rundown of facts about the Anthony Nolan Trust and the National Blood Service. It saves them hours explaining everything, over and over again, to the thousands of well-wishers who turn up at these affairs.

The Letter That Made Carol Cry

Dean and Carol were satisfied that their own do-it-yourself clinics were collecting plenty of new names and samples for the bone marrow registers. But they had their doubts that the official blood clinics were doing their bit. In fact, the couple discovered that the National Blood Service had actually cut down their efforts to recruit bone marrow donors. They were still concerned that new volunteers, would balk at having bone marrow extracted under a general anaesthetic. Worst still, from the couple's point of view, the service had now banned new donors being tested for bone marrow at the same time as they gave blood. Under the new rules, people had to give two lots of blood before their name could be added to the bone marrow list. This meant a delay of six to eight months before a first-time blood donor could expect to join the bone marrow register, precious time that Alice couldn't afford.

Dean and Carol consulted the Barnetts, who confirmed that these constraints on bone marrow volunteers weren't in place during Molly-Ann's campaign. When Paul and Mandy held a clinic, blood donors were also tested for their suitability to give bone marrow. But when Carol asked a senior local representative of the National Blood Service to revert to the old system to give Alice a better chance, he said it couldn't be done.

Following on from their meetings in London, the Maddocks decided to appeal to a higher level. They wrote to the National Blood Service at their headquarters in Colindale, North London, asking that anyone visiting a blood clinic for the first time should be invited to test for bone marrow as well.

When the reply came, Carol was off work, caring for Alice who was again too ill to attend school. The little girl had some familiar symptoms – sharp pains in her legs, nausea and a relentless throbbing ache in her temples. Carol perched on the stairs, going through the second mail as Alice slept fitfully on the sofa in the lounge. Among the bundle was a letter from the National Blood

Service. Carol's heart quickened with anticipation, but as she read, the paper became damp with tears. It was a long letter and it was obvious some trouble had been taken to look closely into Alice's case. But it was a letter that should never have been sent to the parents of a child whose life is in the balance.

The writer, a senior official of the service, had little sympathy with the Maddocks' campaign to register more blood donors. She thought the crusade only put her staff in an impossible position. 'During the last appeal', her letter read, 'members of staff worked considerable amounts of overtime, and some chose to cancel their family holidays, in order to cope with the unprecedented high workload.' She went on, 'We do everything we can, within our means, to enlarge the International Bone Marrow Register, but I consider it unfair to ask our expert staff to do overtime, every time there is an appeal.'

Just as Carol finished reading the letter, the phone rang. It was Margaret Watson at the *Dewsbury Reporter*, making her regular call for news. A shaking Carol read some of the letter to her. Margaret was furious. 'They can't treat you like that!' she cried. On his return from work, Dean was even more infuriated. 'The letter was an outrage,' he said angrily. 'They were trying to turn us into the baddies by saying that our campaigning for Alice was putting their staff under pressure.' He picked up the phone and told me what had happened...

* * *

Next morning, Carol was going to work, Alice was not well enough to attend school, but insisted on going anyway, and Dean was about to return to duty. There was a gentle knock on the front door. Carol tugged back a corner of the lounge curtain and was surprised to see a television crew from Sky News. It was only the beginning. All plans to work were abandoned as a phalanx of TV people came and went all day – the local and national BBC, ITN, Yorkshire TV, CNN, and a few other camera teams the family was too hassled to identify. Reporters who tried to track down the senior director who wrote the letter were told that she was out of the country. I phoned the National Blood Service and was given the same line. But they insisted that the writer was 'certainly not' the kind of person to send offensive letters to parents, and there must be some kind of misunderstanding. 'I bet she regrets sending it now,' I said.

As Dean continued to seethe about the letter, the worst bits were being reproduced in national and local newspapers. The *Daily Mail* carried this headline: 'We're just trying to save our little girl, yet health chiefs say that it's too much trouble'. A leader writer in the *Yorkshire Post* had this to say: 'Dean and Carol's concerns extend beyond their own family. In efforts to help other in similar circumstances, they volunteered to campaign for the National Blood Service. For their trouble they were slapped rudely and hurtfully in the face by the very service supposedly dedicated to life-saving.' The article added: 'This response is unforgivable and barely credible.'

The media coverage was all very critical of the National Blood Service. It may have been a coincidence, but by the end of the week, new machines were wheeled into the department's bone marrow laboratory, making the processing of samples a much faster service. These sophisticated giants could automatically sift through and test volunteers' samples round the clock, seven days a week. The Maddocks were elated. From now on the 'blood lords' would find it much harder to argue that they couldn't cope with an influx of new donors.

The National Blood Service told journalists that now they were automated, their revised target was 15,000 new bone marrow registrations in the coming year, as opposed to 5,000 three years previously. But that compares with 10,000 donations of blood given each and every day. The Maddocks took this news as yet more evidence that blood was the service's priority and the bone marrow register was their 'Cinderella' operation. Not a happy thought, when your daughter's life depends on it.

To give patients a better chance, the couple decided that the best solution was to take responsibility for bone marrow from the National Blood Service altogether and entrust it to an entirely new department. This body would have a management team dedicated to bone marrow and would set bigger targets for the national register. The idea was soon to find favour at the very top, but for now it seemed just another impossible dream.

The Good, the Kind and the Ugly

Alice's website is crammed with emails from people anxious to support the family. A familiar theme is 'never give up'. The advice is superfluous because the Maddocks never will. They constantly remind themselves that Alice's saviour is only one phone call away. Their sustaining thought is that she needs just one person with the right match to join the register. They know that happy endings to the bone marrow search happen all the time. There is no typical donor. They walk all the different corridors of life. But let's take just one example to tempt you to put your own name down...

Keith Butler mends railway tracks in and around Haverfordwest in south-west Wales. Aged 44, he's married to Pearl. They have a twelve-year-old son, Karl. Not long after registering, Keith was contacted because his bone marrow was found to match that of a 30-year-old man in Germany. After failing to find a suitable donor for this leukaemia patient in his own country, the search turned to Britain. Keith has the rare blood group RhD negative – exactly what the German doctors were looking for. They searched the files of 300,000 possible British donors – and his was the only matching blood group. Keith went into the BUPA Hospital in Cardiff for an operation to remove some of his rare bone marrow. He wasn't exactly cheerful about it, this being his first ever operation.

The doctor who flew over to perform the surgery, rushed back to Germany with his prize. Amazingly, he was able to supervise the life-giving transplant for his patient later on the same day. Back in Wales, Keith was a bit bruised and sore for a week or two, but overjoyed to have saved a life. 'I feel fit as a fiddle – and very glad I went through with it.' Keith now recruits many friends, relatives, neighbours and workmates to give bone marrow.

Keith Butler's generous act backs up the Maddocks' complaint that too little is done to make blood donors aware that their bone marrow is just as welcome as their blood. Keith gave blood for more than eight years before he picked up a leaflet on bone marrow at a

donor clinic run by his local council. Then he waited another
eighteen months before a medical examination was arranged by the
National Blood Service to give his marrow the all clear. Dean and
Carol regard that as a ridiculous delay for patients who urgently
need marrow now.

* * *

Not everyone on the bone marrow lists is as altruistic as Keith
Butler. There's a certain kind of donor who brings fear to the
patients and their families who pin all their hopes on the register.
They're supposed to be on the list to help anyone who needs their
marrow – but when it comes to the crunch, this type of donor will
only give for somebody they know. The desire to save one
individual, and nobody else, isn't rare. A man who left a message on
Alice's website caused a wave of indignation in Dean and Carol. 'I
want to know if I am a match for Alice's marrow. I only want to do
it for Alice. I am not interested in a global register. Where do I go
from here?'

Carol felt like telling him in crude terms, but she gritted her teeth
and posted a polite reply. 'You can't register for just one person.
Please reconsider – and add your name to the general register. Your
marrow could be the exact match to save Alice's life.'

She thought the man's email was offensive. She wondered why
anyone should be prepared to offer his or her bone marrow only to
Alice and yet decline to help anyone else. Alice was a complete
stranger. The offer showed the man was not selfish and could be
moved by Alice's predicament. But why exclude other patients?
Was there a racial undertone to this, she wondered? Or even a daft
objection to saving someone of a different religion? The fact that the
message-poster had said he didn't want to join a global register,
suggested some kind of xenophobia. But whatever the reason, Carol
was grieved by it.

This all-for-one and not-for-all mentality leads to harrowing
tragedies of the worst sort. Most parents in West Yorkshire with a
child needing that vital bone marrow match, are saddened at what
happened to a cheerful, boisterous eight-year-old leukaemia
patient called Jack Gails. He had had leukaemia since he was

three. At one time, the Anthony Nolan Trust could only stage
special clinics if parents threw themselves into fund-raising and
collected £5,000. Jack's parents, Kate and Peter, were dedicated
crusaders and had done this four times. One day, it seemed their
efforts were rewarded. 'Dr Mike' told them a match had been
found for Jack on the register. The donor was approached and
went through the first stages of giving marrow. But then
inexplicably he changed his mind. He simply declined to help. He
knew the implications of a refusal, but that's what he did. Jack's
mother Kate doesn't know if attempts were made to persuade him
to think again – it's not policy to give details, she was told. She
was never given any information at all. But whatever the reason
for this seemingly shameful choice, Jack, a natural joker, always
smiling, with his freckles and short spiky hair, was denied his
only chance of life.

For the final few precious days, Jack stayed in his parents'
bedroom. He said he wanted to go bowling, but of course he
couldn't. Kate and Peter tucked him in their bed and cuddled him.
They were still gently holding him as, sedated by morphine, he
passed peacefully away. His mother said he didn't know he was
dying, but he was aware 'something was different'. He wasn't
unhappy when that something different did happen. He was buried
in his favourite 'Action Man' jeans and his fashionable hooded top.
Kate 'wept and wept and wept'.

Later she did a brave interview for local television. You might
expect her to tear angrily into the potential donor whose callous
decision had cost her son his life. But she didn't. Instead, she praised
Jack's life and the eight happy years he'd given to his family and
friends. 'For a few weeks afterwards we tried to understand what
might have been going through that person's mind,' she said. 'I was
bewildered by it. But ever since then I have done all I can to squeeze
it out of my mind. All I know is that Jack was a wonderful child, not
a saint, a real boy and sometimes rather naughty, but loving and
kind. We miss him so much.'

Typically, Dean tried to understand, too. 'A lot of people don't
think about what they're doing, they just go along with the flow.

Maybe friends pressure them into doing things. It's hard to fathom how anyone could make a refusal that leads to the death of a child, but that's human nature. We can't change it.'

* * *

But for every depressing story like that, there are dozens with a happy ending. The great majority of people who sign up to give parts of themselves to help others are as altruistic as you would expect. In Wilsden, near Bradford, Joanne Town, a champion squash player, heard about a local girl of Alice's age, who also needed a bone marrow transplant. She decided to give a sample. It didn't match the girl, but three years later, she got a call. Would she go immediately to University College Hospital in London where her exact marrow type was needed to save a patient's life? Joanne was mightily disappointed. The call couldn't have come at a worse time for the 34-year-old champion. She'd been training all year to try to take a hat trick of titles at a big squash tournament in Leeds. But the dates clashed. So when she should have been achieving a life-long ambition of sporting glory, Joanna was lying face down in an operating theatre, as bone marrow was syringed from her back. She said afterwards, 'It was tough. But really there was no decision to be made.'

There's little doubt that there would be many more names on Britain's two registers if giving bone marrow were as straightforward as giving blood. A blood donation is as simple as having a needle put in your arm. But bone marrow volunteers must be prepared for a 48-hour stay in hospital. They're given a general anaesthetic and wheeled into an operating theatre. A surgeon inserts a needle into the hip bone and the marrow is sucked out. Patients feel sore when they come round. It sounds onerous, but of course the procedure pales to nothing, compared to the inner glow of saving a life. Donors say this is the most satisfying feeling of them all.

Going on the register doesn't necessarily mean you will be called. But if your marrow does match a patient almost anywhere in the world, you'll be expected to give up whatever you're doing and rush into a hospital immediately.

Alice's Election

MPs are very sensitive to health controversies before a general election. The 2001 election was no exception. Health and education are the two issues most favoured by the press. So we thought it would be a good idea to push Alice's case back into the headlines somewhere in the middle of the election build-up, a time when new stories are thin on the ground. Alice's tale – and the lack of resources holding back the number of bone narrow donors – might provoke a hurried pre-election promise from the Labour government. But as Labour MPs were hardly likely to criticise their own record in power, it was probably up to the opposition to do the provoking.

The Tory's Shadow Health Minister Liam Fox had already been involved in Alice's story (when the National Blood Service was criticised for asking the Maddocks not to campaign for more donors). So this seemed a good place to start. I rang the Conservative headquarters about three weeks before polling day. At first they seemed interested. Somebody took a few notes and I was told their top PR person would ring back. But he never did. I made a few more follow-up calls, but you learn to recognise a brick wall in this business.

That left the Liberal Democrats. A party worker seemed enthusiastic. She said it sounded a very good topic for them and they would look into Alice's case. But after a week's waiting, I rang back and found they hadn't done anything whatsoever. Exasperated, I found out where their health spokesman was based and twice phoned his campaign office, suggesting he got in touch. I was quite insistent with the party worker who answered the call, but they seemed very busy and I'm not sure the message was passed on. Anyway there was no response.

Some months after the election, the Lib Dems finally woke up to Alice. One of their researchers phoned, saying the party now had a new spokesman on health who was very interested in her story. Would the family welcome a call from him to see if he could help?

I rejected the offer. As Labour was now firmly back in power, I was reluctant to turn Alice into a political football. It would be a long time, I reasoned, before a Lib Dem MP would have any real influence on events. In retrospect, this was a stupid decision, influenced by irritation that the party hadn't helped when it really mattered. I should have embraced their assistance. At worst, it wouldn't have done any harm.

Though the Maddocks' experiences plainly made a strong stick to beat the government with, the main opposition parties failed to grab it and I gave up on both of them. I began to think the general election was of no use to Alice. As you'll see later, I was utterly wrong.

Despite my disillusionment, Dean and Carol still thought the general election was fertile ground to stir up some interest. They pressed me to think of something else. There was, I decided, another way to make the Cabinet squirm...

The *Today* Incident

Until now, the thrust of Alice's newspaper, radio and television campaign was to rope in more donors by bringing her illness to the notice of ordinary people. But Dean and Carol were just as anxious to chivvy the National Blood Service to do some more serious recruiting themselves. They also wanted substantial funds to be pumped into the process. As a government department, the National Blood Service is subject to pressure from health ministers and, to a lesser extent, run-of-the-mill members of parliament. But how could Alice's fight for health be brought to the attention of MPs? Anybody who knows about broadcasting has the answer to that.

BBC Radio Four's *Today* programme goes out at breakfast time to more decision-makers than any other radio or television show in Britain. It's keenly listened to by Cabinet ministers, anxious to pick up criticisms of themselves, so they can act quickly to nip any embarrassment in the bud. The programme also provides an easy source for politicians looking for instant issues to expound – and so enhance their reputations.

Having previously done time as a reporter on *Today*, I was aware how strong a magnet the programme is to anyone with influence, and not just MPs. It was high time the Alice Maddocks story was aired by its celebrated presenter John Humphrys. I knew that a simple appeal for more resources for the blood service wouldn't attract the hard-nosed editors of *Today*. What was needed was a whiff of controversy. The Maddocks were convinced the National Blood Service wasn't doing enough to find bone marrow donors. But they insisted they were. Potential for a lively radio exchange, I thought.

Most people who ring national radio programmes don't get very far. They're usually referred to the BBC website or asked to write in. But I still had my old BBC staff number. Rather like the service number allocated to soldiers, it's something you never forget. I quoted it to the switchboard in my 'member of staff' voice and asked for *Today*'s 'forward planning department'. There used to be a planning office when I worked there, and nothing much changes at the BBC.

The *Today* producer who answered was keenly interested. I gave her the number of the National Blood Service in West Yorkshire, so they could arrange an interview with one of their directors at the same time. Half an hour later, Dean phoned to say arrangements had been made for both he and Carol to call at Radio Leeds, ten miles from home. From there they would be linked to the *Today* studio in London.

Later that afternoon, the arrangements collapsed. Carol rang to say that a film about Alice had just appeared on ITV. Producers of Esther Rantzen's *That's Esther* picked that day to feature Alice's illness and her need for a donor. It showed Chloe and Alice sharing their garden swing. Someone on the *Today* programme had seen it, and a senior producer rang Carol to say everything was off; they didn't want to run a story just aired by a rival broadcaster. Carol was distraught. She couldn't understand why the need to be first is so important to journalists. Do it better, yes. But why first?

'Don't worry,' I said, sounding more confident than I felt. 'Keep practising what you want to say. You're still on the radio.' I quickly phoned *Today*. A courteous voice told me they were sorry, but weren't prepared to repeat something they'd just seen on ITV. Trying not to sound indignant, I argued that *Today* was being offered a live debate between the parents of a dying child and a prominent representative of the blood service, whom they alleged were letting them down. It was good stuff, real human interest, a lively debate and so on. But I knew I wasn't getting anywhere.

Yet all wasn't lost. The silver principle when dealing with radio and TV shows – and in fact, dealing with any organisation at all – is, if at first you don't succeed, go to the top. I put down the phone, waited half an hour, dialled again, and asked for *Today*'s supremo, Rod Liddle. He wasn't there, but Juliette Dwyer, the deputy editor, was.

She seemed prepared to listen. While I spoke, there were no interruptions but neither were there any grunts of agreement. This was disconcerting, but I pressed on. Why were they pulling the story, just because a 'soft' piece on Alice had just appeared on ITV? The press and TV had already covered that aspect of Alice's story, but the *Today* programme was being offered something quite different: an exclusive debate over whether the National Blood Service had enough resources to save children like Alice. The fact that Alice had appeared on ITV in a piece solely about her illness wouldn't matter to the public.

'Well, it matters to us,' replied the deputy editor, breaking her silence.

'Yes, but what we're giving you is an important follow-up to a story that is widely known. This is an exclusive angle. And anyway, you know the *Today* audience is quite different to the one watching ITV on a Sunday lunchtime.'

I sensed I was losing her. Something else was needed to change her mind. So I resorted to a tactic that often worked in promoting the Maddocks – undiluted emotional blackmail. 'Look, there's a chance to do something really useful with your programme here. The couple are counting on this interview. They're in this terrible position of trying to save their little girl's life. They are extremely vulnerable and under stress, and you really shouldn't be treating them this way.'

I piled it on a bit more. 'You said you would do it and you really can't reject them now. Especially for the trivial reason that they helped with a different kind of film the day before, in a television slot that was hardly peak viewing time. This is very upsetting for them.'

Juliette Dwyer probably thought I was going over the top. But she surprised me when she said, 'All right, we'll go ahead.' Completely thrown by this ready agreement, I mumbled thanks and hung up before she changed her mind. It was a mature choice which programme chiefs sadly don't always make. In my experience, many of them stubbornly stick to their original decisions, if only to save face. But this time, professionalism held court. The producer did a U-turn because she accepted the arguments – or perhaps she just wanted, in a small way, to help prevent the death of a princess.

* * *

The arrangements were reinstated, with one exception. Alice was feeling unwell and back in hospital. Carol stayed at her bedside, while Dean got up at 6 a.m. and made his way rather nervously, into the Leeds studio.

It was the programme's most popular presenter, John Humphrys who conducted the interview. He sounded extremely sympathetic. Dean, quietly spoken and confident, gave careful, well-considered answers. In the other corner, representing the National Blood Service was their national spokeswoman, Dr Angela Robinson. She answered calmly, politely putting the Blood Service's view that they were doing all they could, and that nobody could expect more of them. It was not a bloody and violent battle of the airwaves. Dean is too reserved for that, and Dr Robinson stayed cool and calm. It was Dean who squeezed in the last word though, claiming emphatically that the service should be doing much more to swell the donor register.

Listening in bed, I thought Dr Robinson fielded the arguments pretty well: you can't really win when you oppose the father of a little girl whose life is on a knife edge. However, Dean struck just the right note as a quietly concerned father and firing the last salvo of the debate did the trick. The interview couldn't have been better timed – immediately after the seven o' clock news, when ministers, MP's and the country's decision-makers are browning the toast. Satisfied that Dean had once again made the most of his opportunities, I rolled over and went back to sleep, the noisy breakers of Carmarthen Bay fading away in my head.

By now, Dean and Carol were well satisfied with the mountain of appeals for donors that had featured in newspapers and on radio and TV. The tally of articles and appearances far exceeded those for Molly-Ann Barnett, and she'd found two matching donors, making her well again. Even so, the press interest so far, was nothing compared to the coverage sparked by a cascade of extraordinary events yet to come.

Carol's Obsession with Another Man

Carol could think of no blacker indictment of the Government's stewardship of Britain's health than that children are dying because there's not enough money to register more bone marrow donors. But did the Prime Minister even know about the problem? She suspected not. She wrote a letter to Downing Street:

> We write to you with a desperate plea for help. Our daughter has a right to a full and healthy life as set out in the Human Rights Act and the Children's Act. It should not be impaired due to lack of finances. We feel it's not our responsibility to campaign for new bone marrow donors. Despite all our efforts, we know that a great deal more could be done in helping us find a donor for Alice.

Please, please take action to make positive changes for the future, not only for Alice but for all those in need.

Like most people who write to the Prime Minister, Carol expected the letter to be read by him. But as thousands of letters are addressed to Number 10 every week, that rarely happens. The bland reply they received from a Downing Street assistant, a week later, was discouraging. 'The Prime Minister has asked me to arrange for a minister in the Department of Health to reply to you directly.'

Tony Blair was yet to find that when Carol and Dean Maddocks approach someone, they expect him to do something about it – even if that person is busy governing Britain. He was to learn this fact in a very public and embarrassing way in about two months' time. But for now, the Maddocks just gave the Prime Minister a foretaste of their extraordinary determination. They were irritated by the way their letter was shuffled across to an underling in the Health Department and they fired off another letter to Number 10. This time the couple uncharacteristically dropped their civility. They couched their disappointment in acrid terms.

We wrote to you in the hope you would back our campaign. We then received a reply saying the details would be passed onto the Department of Health.

If we'd thought the Department of Health would do something, we would have written to them!

[The tone became even harsher.] Time and time again we see you on television pledging extra cash for the health service and this month you went on record with: 'Not one person should be denied the chance of life.'

Well, between the Health Service and the National Blood Service, Alice is being denied the 'Chance of life'. Please act immediately. Time is running out for Alice. Make a commitment, NOW...'

Yours sincerely
Dean and Carol Maddocks

* * *

Pupils in class 3 at Alice's village school also felt Mr Blair should be doing something to help. Encouraged by their acting head teacher, Craig Batley, they wrote 28 letters begging the Prime Minister to intervene. This one is from eight-year-old Abigail Dickinson, 'Alice helps class 3 and likes tidying up. She makes sure everybody is all right. She cannot play or do PE, because she can run out of breath very easily. She needs bone marrow. Please help her.' Another classmate, Edward Brackstone wrote, 'I'm sorry to say Alice is poorly. I know you are busy but try to help Alice. She helps other children. She is nice and good.'

Grateful though she was for the school's efforts to engage Mr Blair's attention, Carol suspected people around him were avoiding further demands on his time by stopping the message from getting through. She was convinced that if she cut out the middlemen and told Tony Blair to his face about Alice, he would be appalled by Britain's small total of bone marrow recruits and would divert money into the service. True, in her more sensible moments, this aim seemed a wild fantasy, but she would try, anyway.

The general election was getting ever nearer and by then the Prime Minister was making whistle stops all over the country on a fatiguing campaign trail. For security reasons, his walkabouts were kept secret from the public. But Carol suspected that news editors would have been told exactly where he would turn up, so his vote-catching speeches could make the papers. She dialled journalists who'd shot film on Alice for both Yorkshire Television and the BBC's local *Look North* programme. She also contacted everyone she knew on the regional press.

Carol had met enough journalists to know that when you want to learn something not likely to be volunteered freely, you never ask a direct question. So she simply chatted to journalists on the pretext of letting them know how Alice was bearing up. Her ploy worked. During a long, rambling phone call, somebody let it slip that the Prime Minister was about to visit a certain York hospital. This was it! Her chance to force her way through the crowds and tell Mr Blair all about Alice. She would go on and on at him, shouting, refusing to shut up, until he agreed to help. Cameras would be there, and the world would either hear his hurried promises or brutally criticise his refusal to help. She was relishing a very public row.

But the Maddocks' fickle luck turned against her. At short notice, Alice suddenly needed a blood transfusion on the very day of Mr Blair's visit to York. The couple had vowed that whatever else happened, Alice's treatment would always have top priority. So, spitting feathers, Carol reluctantly gave up her plan to make the 80-mile round trip. Still, that failure to challenge the Prime Minister only fired up her grim resolution to bring Alice's case to his notice. Though it was an unlikely aspiration, it was eventually to come off, preserving the lives of hundreds of people, mostly children.

Determined though they were to bring the bone marrow crisis directly to Mr Blair's attention, the couple were now stumped on how to proceed. Apart from writing another letter, which seemed pointless, what could they possibly do? But it wasn't long before they knew exactly how to move on. Once again the encroaching general election opened the door...

* * *

As usual, attempts were made by broadcasting barons to persuade leaders of the main political parties to slug it out in an American-style live television debate. As usual, the programme chiefs failed. But this time there was a compromise. The three leaders agreed to take part in a special edition of *Question Time*, BBC Television's prime-time current affairs audience show. They would be questioned not by each other, but by the audience. At the end of an earlier programme, a telephone number was given for viewers to call if they wanted to be part of Mr Blair's grilling, scheduled just eight days before polling day. Carol left a hopeful message on *Question Time*'s answerphone. When a researcher rang back, Carol told her all about Alice and said she'd like to tackle the Prime Minister on the shortage of bone marrow donors. It worked. She and Dean were invited to join in the big broadcast, though a mighty snag arose.

Since writing her first story on Alice, Margaret Watson of the *Dewsbury Reporter* rang the Maddocks at least once a week to keep the story bubbling along. During one of their chats, Carol mentioned she was to appear on *Question Time* with Tony Blair. The paper printed the story a month before the programme. Northern correspondents on the *Sun* spotted the article and made a note in the news diary. Three weeks later, on the eve of the big election show, a *Sun* reporter rang Carol. She was cautious about speaking to the press about their appearance on *Question Time*. She did not want to be accused of colluding with the media. Nevertheless, she told him exactly what she would ask Mr Blair if she were chosen to do so but rather hoped he would not put it to print.

However, the story was given a big splash on page 7 alongside an article by the man himself, Tony Blair: 'The parents of a dying girl will confront Tony Blair live on TV tonight – to ask why she can't get a life-saving bone marrow transplant.' The story under the headline read: 'The NHS donor register has not been able to find a match. Mum Carol and dad Dean will grill the PM on BBC 1's *Question Time*.' Dean was also quoted, 'One way or another we intend to get answers from Mr Blair.'

The couple were anxious about this publicity; however, it just might help find the donor they needed. Millions more people would be aware that Carol was hoping to confront the Prime Minister that night. They would tune in, agree with her, and volunteer to become donors. But if they expected the producers of *Question Time* to be pleased with the *Sun*'s free plug, they were wrong. This became painfully clear later in the day...

The Mandarin and the Pirate

The American pirate Captain John Paul Jones used to anchor his eighteen-gun sloop of war *Ranger* off Caldey Island. He cunningly chose a bay on the south side, to be hidden from the mainland. The few inhabitants of this tiny sliver of land, off the south-west coast of Wales, were used to seeing the skull and cross bones on visiting ships. In fact, they made quite a nice living out of supplying dubious vessels with fresh beef from their celebrated herds. Two hundred and twenty-five years later, on a blistering June day, ferryman Graham Waring steered his boat into a jetty on Caldey Island. Cutting the engine, he glided in with his cargo of holidaymakers from the nearby seaside resort of Tenby.

Suddenly, the sultry air was filled with an alien electric sound mocking the summer peace. I was a passenger in the boat and Graham called out to me, 'You've got a message on your bleeper.' I glanced at the old-fashioned pager I use to isolate me from the mobile phones of every Tom, Dick and Harry. The message was: 'Please ring Mark Damazar at the BBC.' Caldey Island is home to Cistercian monks who have no interest in material progress. Consequently, time has passed it by. There is a public phone by the 1940s-style post office. But the message said nothing about any urgency, so I didn't ring back until I was back in Tenby three hours later. Mark Damazar is deputy director of BBC News. He was also involved in that night's crucial production of *Question Time*.

Damazar began politely enough, but something in the tone warned me this wouldn't be pleasant. I was right. 'I'm very disappointed that you told the *Sun* newspaper that Mrs Maddocks is to ask a question of Mr Blair tonight. This puts us in a very difficult position. We have *Question Time*'s integrity to consider.' He went on to say that questions were always taken from the studio audience on a random basis. Sometimes people succeeded in asking a question, sometimes they didn't. The *Sun* article said Carol would definitely ask a question. This made it appear that those members of the audience singled out by David Dimbleby were planted. This, said the BBC executive, sternly was never the case. Mark Damazar was controlled and courteous, but his voice was cold. He seemed very affronted. I had a nasty feeling that the Maddocks would probably be kicked off tonight's show.

Having heard the BBC executive out, I suggested that he was wrong. I had not told the *Sun* the Maddocks would have a go at Tony Blair on *Question Time*. Although I could easily have amassed some pre-programme publicity that way, I hadn't alerted one paper to

Carol's appearance. Not in deference to the BBC, but because the media impact would be even stronger after the event.

I explained to Mark that the Maddocks' local newspaper had a running campaign to find a donor for Alice. Every week, a reporter rang for news to keep the crusade boiling. Carol had been so excited by her chance to put Alice's plight directly to Tony Blair that she'd told the *Dewsbury Reporter* all about it. That was natural enough, surely? And anyway, though she'd spoken at length to the BBC, nobody warned her off the press.

I turned up the pressure. 'You have to remember, Mark, that Mr and Mrs Maddocks are not part of the media. They're thrilled by an opportunity to talk to the Prime Minister about their daughter. They've tried very hard for that chance, long before Mr Blair agreed to go on *Question Time*. They see nothing wrong with passing on their good news to their local paper. Why shouldn't they?'

Damazar softened then. 'I won't keep them off the programme. In fact, that was never our intention. But they must take their chances with everyone else. Remember that most people in the audience don't get a chance to ask anything.'

He assured me that the presenter David Dimbleby would not have been shown the *Sun* newspaper by the production team. And even if he saw the article in passing, he was too professional to be influenced by it. It would not prevent him from taking a question from the Maddocks. But neither would it encourage him to do so.

* * *

I still had my doubts, though. I felt the Maddocks might be deliberately ignored now. Perhaps the Labour party would ring the BBC and insist that a question from the Maddocks be blocked. On the other hand, now the Prime Minister had been forewarned, Labour's media department might actively push for it to be included. After all, Mr Blair (or his spin doctors) now had the time to prepare a snappy, well-informed answer to put himself in a rosy light.

Then again, any pressure to include the Maddocks might have the opposite effect – the BBC could, and probably would, take umbrage at being asked to include material pushed at them by New Labour.

A very good reason why the BBC might want to include the Maddocks in the show also passed through my mind. The producers of *Any Questions* were aware that Britain's journalists would be scrutinising the programme for a tasty story to print or broadcast afterwards. Almost certainly, a wrong move by the Prime Minister would give birth to big headlines the next day. The Maddocks were obviously gunning for the Prime Minister. Accept a question from them, and there would be useful publicity pickings for the BBC.

As I talked to Damazar on the phone, yet another thought struck me. If Dimbleby didn't pick out the Maddocks, the BBC could be accused of trying to protect the Prime Minister. The *Sun* had asserted that Carol would definitely ask her question and to deny her chance on the night could make it look like a case of second thoughts.

This was beginning to make my head ache, but the many ramifications of the situation continued to pour through my brain. If David Dimbleby had seen the *Sun* article – and it was hard to imagine his not reading the papers carefully before the show – how could he stay unbiased? Surely, he would be looking out for guests who would promote a lively exchange with the Prime Minister and so brighten the programme.

But the Corporation's news chief, Mark Damazar was still on the phone and it was now time for our secret weapon – a bit more emotional blackmail. 'I would hope that you give the Maddocks every consideration when they arrive. They have enough on their plate, without extra pressures. I'm sure you'll be kind to them because we all have to appreciate that all they're trying to do is to save their little girl's life.' He promised that of course they would receive every courtesy.

Even so, it was with trepidation that I phoned Dean to tell him about the BBC's displeasure. He was perturbed by the news, so I quickly assured him that it didn't really matter. They'd had an assurance from high in the BBC that the article would have no bearing on their chances of asking Mr Blair their question. But given what had happened, the couple now needed as much help as they could get.

To shorten the odds of being invited to confront Mr Blair, I regurgitated some trade secrets for getting on television. To stand out in the audience, I advised them to put on clothes of the same bright colour, the more garish the better. They shouldn't wear striped or checked clothes because they 'strobe' – that is, jump around on the screen. They should sit bolt upright in their seats to make them appear taller, and therefore more important. And they shouldn't hold handbags, pens, spectacles or other objects that might be construed as a distraction by the director.

I also advised them what to do once they were picked out. They should not just ask a question and sit down, but should make lots of comments, too. These remarks should come before the actual query, not after it, because the couple wouldn't be cut off until their question had finished. They should speak quickly with no 'ums' and 'ers', and avoid any gaps between sentences. The slightest hesitation would make it easy for David Dimbleby to nip in and silence them. Finally I pointed out a handy psychological ploy – the longer people are able to speak without interruption, the less likely they are to get a brief answer.

I wished them luck and then, because I wasn't really expecting their question to be aired at all – and couldn't bear to watch for an hour, willing this to happen – I decided to go to bed early that night.

Meanwhile, Dean and Carol prepared for what they knew was the most important TV appearance they'd ever make in the fight for Alice. And yet there was no guarantee they would be given the Prime Minister's ear. All they could be sure of, after my phone call from the BBC, was that they had no priority to speak to Mr Blair, possibly even the reverse.

* * *

Question Time had taken over a sports hall in Milton Keynes for the people's debate with the Prime Minister. At lunchtime, the pair set off for the venue in Dean's Renault Mega. They were uneasy about leaving home at all. Not because they were nervous about appearing on *Question Time* (they were, after all, television veterans by now) but they didn't want to leave Alice's side. She was unwell again, suffering headaches, pains in her joints and a high temperature after another grinding round of hospital treatment.

A warning rattled around Dean's head as he drove towards the northern end of the M1. 'This is a massive opportunity. We have to make the most of it. It's our one big chance to get our message across.' The responsibility seemed enormous to him. 'If we play it right, we could be talking to Tony Blair, the most powerful person in the kingdom.'

The persistent voice in his head grew even stronger. 'Everybody else we've approached in the bone marrow field could easily say, "Well, if it was up to me, I would do anything you ask – but it's not up to me. So I can't help." But Mr Blair is the man at the top. He can't say the decision doesn't rest with me. The buck stops with him.'

The couple were also keenly aware of a tantalising bonus waiting for them if they could pull it off. Bags of newspaper stories and big television interviews would follow a confrontation with the Prime Minister – later tonight and next day. In fact, the more they thought about this big adventure, the higher the stakes seemed to climb.

The uncertainty of the outcome of the affair made Dean feel they were taking part in some bizarre quiz show. 'Would we win the holiday or not? If we didn't, we'd slink out of that hall in Milton Keynes and, feeling unloved and forgotten, drive home to obscurity. On game shows, nobody cares about the losers – and then what would happen to Alice?'

Thinking ahead as usual, Carol had taken an overnight bag in case they had to stay in a hotel and do interviews in the morning. As she packed a second set of smart clothes, she vowed to herself she would definitely need them; she would put Mr Blair on the spot. Nobody was going to stop her. She could not afford to let them. She had a duty to Alice and to the world. At this early stage of the business, she was entirely determined. But this is real life, not a novel. And as usual in real life, her mood passed. Doubts began to sidle up, as they did with Dean on that long journey south. The mission seemed too reliant on chance, perched on a feather, too precarious by half. There would be hundreds of people in the audience all anxious to tackle the Prime Minister. The BBC was already wary of the Maddocks clan. They had no chance.

There were two mobile phones in the car. They switched them on to receive any messages about Alice's health and hear good luck wishes from friends and relatives. Both phones started bleeping as they pulled out of their gravel drive in Hanging Heaton and continued almost non-stop during 150 busy miles to Milton Keynes. But it wasn't friends and relations who were calling. The hungry media were on their trail again. With Dean occasionally prompting at the wheel, Carol fielded questions from newspaper reporters who wanted something on tonight's show. There was no doubt these journalists expected the producers to make sure they got a question in to Mr Blair. Surely the BBC could appreciate a good story! Carol also gave dozens of local and national radio interviews as the car sped through the sweltering afternoon. Balanced on her knees was a desk diary. A succession of callers was keen to arrange interviews the minute the show closed. Others wanted the couple to fill prime slots the following morning. Carol was juggling names and places to fit in as many interviews as she could. This was a daunting chore, as the various TV breakfast shows are miles apart, and there was London's rush hour to worry about too.

The big complication was the fact that the couple were not guaranteed an audience with Tony Blair. Carol never tells lies, but was learning that there are some things you should keep quiet about when talking to reporters. Accordingly she let the hacks assume the Maddocks would definitely set *Question Time* alight.

Though it was a beautiful early summer evening, all was not well in the car. The couple were becoming agitated. The vast number of media requests eventually overwhelmed Carol. Some calls weren't answered. A few interviewers were double-booked in the diary. Dean was so preoccupied with what they hoped to tell Mr Blair that he took wrong turnings, adding precious minutes to the journey. They became ratty with each other as both began to despair of their vital mission. They were sure now they would let Alice down. Failure was inevitable. Abject failure, which they would always regret.

* * *

Much later than they intended, the Renault slipped into the car park of the sports hall at Milton Keynes. Dean and Carol risked their modesty by changing in the car from their travelling clothes of jeans and T-shirts into the smart, vividly coloured clothes they hoped would catch the presenter's eye. A couple of frantic minutes later, dazed, flustered, nervous, and overawed by what they had to do, they joined the rest of a seemingly vast and good-humoured audience. Dean thought there must be at least 400 people there. A frosty feeling assailed his stomach. This wasn't going to work out. Mathematics would defeat them. He guessed that if each question and answer lasted three minutes (on the conservative side) with an introduction and ending from Dimbleby added on, only about seventeen people would be picked out. That gave odds of 23–1 against. Dean grumbled to Carol that you wouldn't expect a horse to win at that sort of price.

But the programme did provide one certain way of being singled out. If you could write down a provocative question, you might be chosen in advance. This was the producer's method of dividing the debate into separate topics. Each questioner chosen in this way began a new subject. To sort out these lucky sheep from the unlucky goats, everyone was asked to write down a starter question, of less than 30 words, on a small white card. Only a few of these cards would be picked to kick off a debate on the main issues of taxes, health, the Euro and so on. Dean scribbled away, but had trouble phrasing his question. He actually wrote out several different questions – all longer than requested. Carol was no help. She was in a dither. She had her pen poised over her card, but couldn't think what to put down. 'I had loads of things to say, but the whole thing was just too important for my brain to function properly. I couldn't get my pen into my head.'

When Carol did manage to phrase a question, it was also too wordy, and she failed to condense it. Neither was happy with the fistful of cards they finally handed into a smartly dressed programme assistant. They weren't surprised when their questions weren't picked.

This setback put both Dean and Carol in a bleak frame of mind. They'd made a rotten start. Now only about a dozen people would be selected at random from a big audience. This reduced their chances

to about 33–1. In racing terms, they were rank outsiders. Dean
eventually realised that, as there were two of them, the odds were
really 15–1, but it wasn't much comfort. If only some of the journalists rooting for them out there could somehow twist David
Dimbleby's arm. Meanwhile, Carol's nerves were becoming
seriously frayed. She made several visits to the toilet to check her
make-up.

Though she could eat nothing, they were offered the usual BBC
hospitality of tea or coffee, orange juice and sandwiches. This can
be a pleasant opportunity for the studio audience to shake off their
stagefright by chatting to each other. But Carol and Dean didn't talk
to anyone. They wanted to 'save their strength for the big moment'
– if it ever came. While Dean nibbled an egg sandwich, both were
aware that corners of eyes were watching them. It was clear that
people around them recognised the couple from their many
television appearances and newspaper photos. Some had seen
Carol's picture in the *Sun* that morning. But oddly, nobody tried to
open a conversation. Perhaps they were radiating too much anxiety.

The couple had brought along copies of the letters sent to Mr
Blair by Alice's classmates. They handed a bundle of them to one of
the researchers. But they quickly realised this was a mistake. If
programme staff hadn't already singled them out as the bolshie
couple mentioned in the *Sun*, these innocent letters would certainly
identify them now. Carol and Dean soon noticed a group of BBC
folk huddled in discussion and glancing towards them. One nodded
in their direction. Rightly or wrongly, they suspected they were
under close observation. 'We felt like suspected terrorists,' said
Carol. 'As if I had hand grenades in my pocket.'

Perhaps nobody on the programme staff ever looked at the
Maddocks with anything other than mild interest. Maybe they just
nursed a keen sympathy for Alice's plight, but Carol and Dean
thought they were unwanted and resented in that room. Carol felt
degraded. 'I hate anyone to think badly of me, or anyone else in our
family. I always have done. And the conviction that they were
keeping a careful eye on us, in case we did something naughty, was
so upsetting.'

The feeling of rejection really did make her feel wretched. 'I just wanted to go and tell the staff and everybody in the audience that we're not bad people; that we just want to help Alice who is so vulnerable, and so needy and so full of life. I wanted them to know that I need Alice to grow up and enjoy every bit of her future, just like everybody else. That's what drove us to go on *Question Time*. But to feel despised when we got there – it was all pretty hard to bear.'

But her wrathful thoughts were interrupted. 'Can we all go into the studio, please?' cried a rather jolly producer. A good-natured queue formed and everyone filed into the sports hall. As Dean and Carol moved into the spacious room their spirits suddenly lifted. Was good fortune with them, after all?

* * *

'We were very lucky with our seats,' Dean explained. 'Smack bang in the middle. About four rows up from the front. For the first time I felt we had a fighting chance.' They'd unwittingly taken some of the best seats in the house. From here, it would be impossible for David Dimbleby to miss their hands in the air. They were also very handy for the cameras and the man controlling the overhead microphone. But luckiest of all, Carol found herself sitting immediately in line with the chair soon to be filled by the man who could help Alice more than anybody on the planet.

'I was going to have full eye contact with Mr Blair,' said Carol triumphantly, 'and I knew then that God was helping us that night.' With Dean, she felt a new confidence replacing the day's miserable apprehension. This came with a secret and malicious thought. Perhaps the production staff suspected she had cunningly planned their entrance so this key seat would fall to her automatically. Let them think it! They would never know the dream seat was due to sheer chance, or as Carol would have it, divine intervention.

But the prominence of their position did nothing to kill the butterflies jiggling in Dean's stomach. 'I was very, very nervous, not because we were on television, but because of the enormity of what we had to do.' Carol was also acutely apprehensive. She recalled afterwards, 'Everyone else in that audience was there to ask questions on taxes, immigration, education and so on. Serious things maybe, but nothing that was a matter of life and death to them. But we had to force ourselves onto Mr Blair for a much more important reason – to keep Alice alive. It's no wonder we were like jelly.'

They felt a bit better, though, when Tony Blair took his seat, just a few feet in front of them. If he could appear relaxed, when the future of his government might hinge on his performance, why should they be in a state? Actually, the Prime Minister was too tired to be nervous. He told his audience he'd dashed to the studio after a day of fast electioneering in several marginal constituencies. But there was no more time for small talk. A studio manager did his 'Five, four, three, two, one' routine and the red light clicked on. The programme was about to invade millions of homes.

* * *

At 1 a.m., the telephone rang in my bedroom in Tenby. It was Carol Maddocks. I had already prepared some words of comfort, knowing she put so much store on talking directly to Tony Blair about Alice. She told me what happened and I was shattered...

Question Time

I went downstairs and played the video tape I'd recorded to see what had happened for myself.

The avuncular figure of Rolf Harris in a bright red, short-sleeved shirt, was holding the airwaves just before the Prime Minister's historic broadcast on BBC1 TV. The youngsters who're the main audience for *Animal Hospital* have little in common with the usual worthy viewers of *Question Time*, but programme planners were relying on seductive trails that had promoted the programme over the last few days. The continuity reader said 'So now on BBC 1 ... Challenge the Leader...' This announcement was followed by a jazzy title sequence, featuring short clips of Mr Blair gesturing rather wildly. (This would have puzzled some viewers as this live programme hadn't started yet.) Then presenter David Dimbleby appeared to declare dramatically: 'Tonight...Challenge the leader in *Question Time*. Live from Milton Keynes, the Prime Minister, Tony Blair, faces the voters...'

Viewers could see that the venue was crowded. Often on shows like this, people fail to make use of their invitations for all sorts of reasons and those who do turn up need to be shuffled around to bulk out the audience. Sometimes, technicians and studio staff have been known to fill a few seats. But tonight every place was clearly taken. In fact, some seats appeared to hold more than one person. The familiar *Question Time* desk for four luminaries in front of the seating area was absent. Instead, Mr Blair cut a lonely figure on a simple office swivel chair perched on a small circular platform, so he could swing round to face a questioner anywhere in the vast room.

Wearing a suit in political grey, a white shirt and dark blue tie, with tiny white spots, Mr Blair began the programme suddenly seeming rather nervous. He blinked twice in his brief opening shot, making him look a bit like a startled rabbit. You couldn't blame him for feeling apprehensive. With the general election now only a few days away, if he painted himself into a corner, or even simply appeared rather shifty, then he might just let the Conservatives back into power. It was as scary as that. He was also facing ordinary people, many of whom would want to tear into him for reasons as varied as genuine concern about an issue to the rare chance to impress friends by arguing with the Prime Minister on the box. Mr Blair was aware of what every politician knows – dealing with the general public is more daunting than fending off your parliamentary colleagues or celebrated interviewers.

Before introducing the first questioner, David Dimbleby reminded the audience that: 'Under our usual *Question Time* rules, Mr Blair hasn't been told what questions he's going to be asked.' This opening announcement gave testimony to the deep concern of Mark Damazar about that day's story in the *Sun*. Because of that article, Dimbleby's proud boast was, for once, not entirely true. Mr Blair was definitely aware of the *Sun*'s story about Carol, and therefore knew in advance at least one question he would be asked – if Carol got the chance.

Dimbleby smoothly introduced the first questioner, an advertising executive called Hannah. Reading carefully from a prepared card on her lap, she wanted to know if Labour was insulting the electorate by its recent poster campaign depicting Conservative leader William Hague as Margaret Thatcher. It wasn't a difficult question and it allowed Mr Blair to relax almost immediately. Hannah and the next few questioners dropped politely out of the picture after making their rather tame points and it was left to the presenter to raise some critical follow-up queries on their behalf.

Not long into the election special, the first question came on health. Carol and Dean, already alert and watchful, moved to the edge of their seats. The questioner was a computer consultant who claimed the Government's manifesto pledges on the National Health Service were the same promises made when Labour was elected last time round. 'Why,' he asked stonily, 'should we trust you again?' Mr Blair replied that the pledges of four years ago were modest. The new deal was more ambitious. Now the programme was warming up. It was clear from the answering back Mr Blair was starting to get that the audience was more interested in health care than the issues of poster campaigning and the Euro, which had gone before. In all, four people asked questions on health. Most of them were professionals in the field, including a family doctor and a hospital consultant. Then David Dimbleby, with little over half the programme left to run, moved out of health and into taxes.

Carol and Dean felt the sharp sting of disappointment. It was as if a spear had passed through them. They turned white with frustration, groaning aloud. It seemed their chance to bring Alice's plight directly to the Prime Minister had evaporated in a cloud of steam. They were stunned. Health care had been raised as an issue, had already taken up nearly a third of *Question Time* and had gone. Dean muttered to himself darkly, 'That's it. We've blown it! We're not going to get anywhere now. There'll be no big TV follow up, no radio interviews, nothing.' Both he and Carol felt physically sick. They were shaking with unhappiness. All that effort in writing to the programme; a car drive of 300 miles to Milton Keynes and back; all their high hopes crushed. They'd forfeited valuable time, which could have been spent with their desperately ill daughter. And for what? Nothing at all – just to fill out the studio audience for a television show.

But the moment of despair didn't last long. The couple realised together that *Question Time* wasn't over yet. Where's there's life there's hope! And this was a live programme. Anything could happen and there was still a precious half hour to go. And if there was one thing Carol had learned over the past eighteen months, it was never to give up. Ever. Cogs in her brain started whirring fortified by adrenaline. People were putting up their hands all over the sports hall now. How could she get a question in? She remembered what I'd told her. 'You're on a live programme; they have no control over you. If you make a scene, the producer won't mind. Neither will David Dimbleby. All self-respecting broadcasters welcome a bit of passion. And even if they do object to your making a scene, what of it? They invited you on the show. They know how worried you are about Alice. They can't dictate your behaviour.'

Carol carefully considered standing up without the presenter's permission. Perhaps she could shout across to Mr Blair without being invited. He was sitting near enough. That would be 'passionate'. But could she really risk that? The ploy could backfire; she might appear to the watching world as merely bad mannered, a rude loudmouth. After struggling with the choice for several minutes, she deferred to modesty, deciding to behave herself. But she did have another idea...

As Dimbleby invited more questions on higher taxes, she pushed her hand straight into the air, stretching to get the greatest possible height. Dean turned and stared at his wife in amazement. He tried to catch her eye and failed. Then he nudged her, whispering hoarsely, 'What the hell are you doing? What do you know about tax?'

'That was the most hairy moment of my life, ever,' Dean acknowledged afterwards. 'I thought she'd flipped. I had no idea what she was up to.' But Carol did. She could raise an issue about tax, or any other election topic, and change it into another health question. She didn't have to be subtle about it – just do it. By now, there were even more upraised hands of people all wanting the singular experience of confronting Mr Blair on television.

Carol glanced round at the audience. Her old fears about being disliked, reviled and denigrated surfaced again. 'If my question is taken,' she hesitated, 'all this lot are going to be looking at me. What are they going to think?' Her hand wavered. She was on the point of putting it down. Then she tried a bit of self-deception.

'There's nobody else here,' she lied to herself. 'The room is empty apart from the Prime Minister and me. Yes, it's just him and me. He's just an ordinary man. It's not the Prime Minister at all. There's nobody at home watching. It's not even being televised...'

A property developer now had the floor, treating the audience to the first lively exchange of the evening. The man was trying to score points and the audience warmed to him. This is what they'd come to see – Daniel in the lion's den. Having allowed it to continue for some minutes David Dimbleby was anxious to get away from this persistent debater whom he thought had bitten away at the Prime Minister for long enough. With the cameras still on the man, the calm and collected presenter cast his eye over the audience, searching for the next questioner. Carol, who'd just checked her watch to observe glumly that time was ebbing away, suddenly saw a glimmer of hope. She managed to catch David Dimbleby's roving eye.

'I saw him glance at me. I got eye contact with him and I wouldn't let go. I mouthed the words, "Please...give...me...a... chance..." Meanwhile, the property developer was still trying to floor the Prime Minister. Dimbleby turned swiftly to the audience, spotting, as you couldn't avoid doing in that sea of sombre clothing, a glaring jacket in glorious rose pink. The attractive, raven-haired woman wearing it held her hand high. And Carol Maddocks heard from Dimbleby the best five words of the year. 'The woman in pink, there...'

'It's me!' she thought. At last the chance to bring Alice's quest for life to the Prime Minister himself. Not only that, but millions would be her witness. If she could only wrest a promise of action from him now, he would have to keep it. She had to stay calm. She had to milk the moment. The programme was live; she could not end up on the cutting-room floor. Nothing could stop her. Of course, she still had to give a hard-hitting, convincing, emotional performance and tie Mr Blair down to a personal guarantee to help. But the hard part – being chosen to speak at all – was over. All she had to do now was put a simple question and get the right answer. It was going to be easy. But was it? To her horror, a walloping great obstacle suddenly arose...

The Attack

Carol's over-worked mind had gone quite blank. She couldn't think what she'd come here to say. Inside the shocking pink suit, she was now shaking with raw fear. 'Please, God, put some words in my mouth,' she breathed. 'There's nothing there. I don't know what I'm going to say. I just don't know what I'm going to say.' She waited for the audience's humiliating laughter as she opened her mouth and failed to utter a word. But then something wonderful happened. Perhaps it was her subconscious mind that rushed to help. But anyway, a stream of eloquence rolled calmly off her tongue. She wasn't sure what she was saying, but everyone was taking notice. The big moment had come, and a valiant mother fighting for her child seized it adroitly.

It took Alice Maddocks' name just a second to bring the programme's current subject of taxation back to the shortage of money in the health service, and just a half second more to narrow down the new topic to bone marrow donors. It was a seamless move. A master stroke.

'Mr Blair, if we pay more money on tax, can we then rely on charities not running our NHS, as they are doing? The British Bone Marrow Register relies on charity to fund it every year.'

A few words later, there was an 'OK' off screen as Dimbleby tried, seemingly prematurely, to hurry Carol along. But Tony Blair was looking keenly interested, his eyes narrowed in concentration.

Carol was encouraged. 'Will you make a commitment tonight that you will put some funding into the Bone Marrow Register? Our child desperately needs a bone marrow transplant. She is going to die without that.' And for emphasis, 'Will you make that commitment and help to save her life?'

The audience became attentive, savouring the most powerful story in the programme so far: a little girl whose life might be ended too soon if the Prime Minister didn't give the right answer. They leaned forwards and sideways for a better view. A few people clapped in anticipation. Most wondered how Mr Blair could possibly refuse such a direct and public plea to save Alice.

But his answer was a let-down. 'I can't make a specific commitment on the bone marrow service. I can only make a commitment on the health service spending. I'm sure . . . '

He wasn't going to get away with that. Carol wasn't having any of it. 'No, it's not good enough!' The camera fastened back on her. 'No, Mr Blair,' she repeated, 'it's not good enough. We've heard this time and time again. We've had talks with ministers of health. We've had conversations with MPs. We've tried to work with the NHS. We've had umpteen meetings with the National Blood Service in this country. We shouldn't have to attend those meetings. We should be having time with our family . . . '

Her next few words were drowned out by noisy applause. The staid audience hadn't been too keen to clap any of the previous questioners.

Carol turned up the heat a shade more. 'It should not be down to individuals like us to campaign to get donors on registers. It is not good enough!' Becoming angry now she stabbed a finger in Mr Blair's direction. 'Your government needs to do the campaigning!'

Alone in his living room in Ossett, near Wakefield, Harry Lister, Carol's father, sat up rigid on the sofa. He was shocked to see his daughter's fierce expression on the telly. He wasn't sure she should be talking to the Prime Minister like that. A reserved man, he would never have done anything of the sort himself. But the initial stab of horror turned almost instantly to admiration and pride. 'Good old Carol!' he cried.

Back at the sports hall, David Dimbleby intervened. 'All right, let Mr Blair answer.'

A seemingly slightly amused, but probably rather shaken, Mr Blair replied that his government was trying to campaign for more donors. 'There are three organisations which deal with bone marrow in this country [he was including the separate Welsh blood service here]. In fact we have the third highest number of donors in the world on the registers.' Then he added: 'I don't know if this is the same case I read about in the paper this morning, but as I understand it, they have been trying to find a proper bone marrow donor for your daughter.'

Carol is adept at expressions of suspicious derision and she delivered one now to the Prime Minister. Then she turned her face to Dean and shot him a 'now it's your turn' look. His first few words were lost, as a microphone swung into position over his head. But soon he was heard to grumble, 'They say they're doing a lot of work, but actually they're not. They're just doing the basics week in, week out.'

Carol came back into the fray. Speaking rapidly to make the most of time, she said, 'Blood donors are not aware that they can become bone marrow donors. Half a million new blood donors come on the register every year. We would like to see them canvassed and asked.'

Mr Blair began, 'Can I just...'. This time David Dimbleby interrupted him, telling Carol, 'You've had a good say. It is a specific case...'

But the Prime Minister insisted on saying more. 'It is a specific case, but because it was in the paper today, I did ask for a briefing on what was happening in relation to bone marrow donors. And they do – or so they say to me – actually ask the blood donors whether they would be willing to give bone marrow...'

Dean chipped in: 'They don't...'

The presenter rebuked him. 'I'm sorry, you must let him answer the question,' adding more kindly, 'I know it's very important to you, but you must let him answer the question...'

Then it happened. Mr Blair made a snap decision. It was one the Maddocks were hoping for, but never really expected. He chose there and then to become personally involved in the fight to save Alice. He told the couple, 'I have heard about your individual case. If you would like me to look into it specifically, I would be very happy.'

Most people would have been utterly content with that promise. Dean was. But Carol Maddocks, always ready to go a step further, pressed for more, 'And I would like to spend some time with you – only half an hour.'

Carol the social worker again fixed him with the fierce look she uses to keep wayward children in line. The Prime Minister smiled, and said 'Yes, OK.'

Victory! A thousand white doves rose from the floor and flew outwards towards the ceiling; a hundred top hats twirled in the air. That's how the moment seemed to Dean and Carol. Clapping and laughter filled the hall. The audience had taken Carol to their hearts and Mr Blair had buckled to her demands. The couple leaned back in their chairs, knowing their glorious mission – to bring Alice's case right to the man at the top – had succeeded. It was over.

Back in Wakefield, Dean's 62-year-old mother Joan and father David watched *Question Time* from a small tent. They'd pitched it in the living room by orders of Alice and Chloe. Head poking through the tent flaps, Joan heard the words 'the lady in pink...' She saw Carol stiffen to challenge Mr Blair and her heart jumped. She was nervous for her daughter-in-law and with a mother's insight knew from Dean's face that he was terrified his wife would say the wrong things. Meanwhile, Alice and Chloe yelled 'Go on, Mum! Go on, Mum. Go on Mum!' They both cheered hard when she did just that. And so did Joan, giggling with pride.

* * *

By all standards, it was a staggering achievement: an ordinary man and wife, standing alone, not backed by a charity or pressure group, winning a promise from the Prime Minister, in front of millions of viewers, that he would personally act to try to save their daughter. Despite world affairs and Britain's current economic and other problems, he'd agreed to look into the case of one little girl.

Long afterwards, people working in television asked Carol and Dean how they'd done it. Why hadn't they been overawed by the occasion? How did they dominate the moment? Other questioners on the programme lacked fire in comparison. Alice's parents brought *Question Time* to life, made the programme talked about for weeks – and showed the human side of Tony Blair.

The odds had been against them. They'd not been chosen by the producer before the programme began to ask a question, as some of the audience had. Many people had later waved their hands about to make their own points to the Prime Minister and had stayed unchosen. That part of *Question Time* devoted to health questions had already come and gone. But Carol had skilfully exploited the fact that the programme was live by craftily converting a question on tax to one about bone marrow transplants.

Who could blame the programme producers for feeling put out? A morning paper had said Carole would 'quiz the Prime Minister', though the rules of the *Question Time* forbade any advance knowledge. The Prime Minister had read the article and asked for a briefing on bone marrow donors. He was fully prepared for Carol before she spoke. And though the BBC had depressed the Maddocks by saying they must take their chances of asking a question with everybody else, they had dominated the second half of the programme through sheer force of personality. But if the BBC ever regretted they'd lost control of *Question Time*, then the publicity the programme received, thanks to Carol's tour de force, consoled them. The country's press, television and radio stations, had looked in vain for a big human interest story to bring colour to a boring election build-up and now at last they had it.

After *Question Time*

As the end credits rolled, Dean was euphoric. Staunchly proud of his wife, he wanted to throw his arms round her. But then the moment was overridden by another impulse. He wished he'd brought a couple of paper bags to put over their heads. He now expected fellow members of the audience to accuse them of having been brazen attention-seekers. At the very least, he prepared himself for a universal snub. He looked at the floor at first, then tentatively raised his head to gaze fearfully around him. These people were British. They wouldn't approve of this sort of thing. They'd been guilty of an unseemly outburst towards a very civilised and dignified leader of the nation. But no... he couldn't have been more wrong. People weren't sending them to Coventry. They were hurtling out of their seats and rushing over to congratulate them. A lot of backslapping was going on. They heard 'well done!' over and over again. Unlike their silent reception before the programme, everybody wanted to talk to them.

Dean was astounded. 'People weren't charging over to see the Prime Minister. They were crossing the room in droves to see us. They were so pleased Carol had given Mr Blair both barrels. For the first time since we left home, we didn't feel like outsiders. The whole world was with us now.'

A doctor from the famous Great Ormond Street Children's Hospital was among the first to congratulate the bewildered couple. He thanked them for highlighting the lack of resources for sick children in such an effective way, left his card and pleaded with them to get in touch. A woman called out, 'That told him!' Another 'Bully for you!' Someone else cried: 'Make sure he keeps his promise!

Vaguely, through the crowd of well-wishers, Dean spotted Mr Blair inching quietly away. He seemed to be anxious to leave the hall quickly. Impulsively, Dean cried out to him, 'Don't forget that you promised us a meeting!'

Mr Blair gave a small wave in reply. Carol saw that restrained gesture and thought he looked a little shifty as he acknowledged her husband's cry. Dean had a similar reaction, thinking scornfully, 'Politicians' promises! I just bet it never happens.'

Television news crews waited outside to interview the Maddocks. There were scores of reporters from radio stations and newspapers. To save time, Dean fielded one set of questions, Carol another. With each interview – and the couple had done hundreds by now – Carol was increasingly aware of the importance of a new angle to reporters, and always thought of something new to tell them. She'd prepared something for this occasion weeks ago and she jubilantly spouted it now.

'Mr Blair started his election campaign in a school. He said then that children are the future of the nation. But Alice is not getting the chance to have such a future. And I wanted him to know that.'

Everyone in Carol's large circle of friends and relatives had noticed how cunning she was becoming to save her daughter. Each word she says in public is aimed at adding ammunition in the tussle for Alice's life. Pointing out that Mr Blair had used the needs of children to launch his campaign to stay in power – and that he'd done it in a school – was a stroke of genius. It made it appear that children's welfare was vital to New Labour's election strategy. This was calculated to force Mr Blair's hand: to make him honour his election pledges – by doing even more to help sick children.

The journalists were keen to note down Carol's quote or register it on their micro-recorders. This was now their big election story, easily the best of the entire campaign.

* * *

Feeling rather like The Beatles after a sixties concert, the couple finally jostled their way back to their car. Inside, the two mobile phones continued to sound as reporters tried to interview them in transit, or to arrange television and radio interviews for the morning. But eager for publicity as they were, the couple first wanted to ring home to check on Alice.

As well as their daughter's health, they had another concern about how things were at home. They'd wanted Alice to see the programme

– it's not often your parents talk to the Prime Minister – but they were worried about exactly what Alice might hear. Carol had thought it important to tell Mr Blair the stark truth that Alice would die without an exact marrow match. And she had done. But how would Alice feel when she heard this? It would certainly upset her. It might even cause far-reaching psychological damage. The couple decided the best way to deal with this dilemma was to talk directly to Alice. Dean told her, the day before the programme, that they might have to say on television that she could die unless the right bone marrow donor was found. But added that she was not to worry because her parents were going to make sure the right person was found. Alice didn't even bother to listen properly.

But hearing that you 'might die' on television is more frightening than a familiar chat at the kitchen table. So when Dean and Carol finally dialled home, about two hours after the programme, they were terrified that Carol's explicit plea to Mr Blair would have petrified Alice. But their fear was groundless. One of the first things Alice said when she came to the phone was, 'It's all right about saying I'm dying. It's OK. I know you had to say that.' Dean and Carol marvelled at their daughter's stoical common sense.

* * *

The early morning television company, GMTV, made arrangements for the couple to stay overnight a smart hotel in London at their expense. But Dean had rarely driven in the capital. They were also disturbed by their mobile phones, which kept bleeping out requests for interviews. By now the couple's nerves were in rags. They were very tired. They'd driven long distances, been pestered by media fixers all day and night, and had undergone a live television ordeal more tense and draining than anyone could be expected to bear. After losing their way several times, they finally pulled into the hotel car park at about 2 a.m.

While the couple slept, national papers and local dailies were having a field day. The *Daily Mail*'s headline over a full-page feature was: 'IT ISN'T GOOD ENOUGH, A SICK GIRL'S PARENTS TELL THE PREMIER'.

Next to a huge picture of Dean and Carol, with a smiling Alice on
mum's knee, the article proclaimed: 'Carol Maddocks asked the
toughest questions he faced on BBC1's Question Time.'

The Maddocks' local newspaper, the *Yorkshire Evening Post*, had
as its front-page lead: 'NOT GOOD ENOUGH, MR BLAIR',
followed by: 'Mum blasts Prime Minister on TV'. The paper also
carried a picture of Carol, taken directly from a television screen,
wearing the fierce 'Carol Maddocks look'. Even her own family
were scared by it.

The newspapers were to refer to the *Question Time* confrontation
for weeks to come. They commended the couple's 'stubborn
inspiration' and 'bravura performance'. Recalling the encounter a
month afterwards, the *Sunday Telegraph* said the couple
'...shrewdly spotted a means of forcing Mr Blair's hand'.

A leader writer in the *Yorkshire Post* said, 'This was a rare,
unscripted and embarrassing moment for Mr Blair on what was
otherwise a carefully stage-managed campaign trail.'

Writing in the *Sunday Telegraph*, the deputy editor Matthew
d'Ancona praised Dean and Carol's 'lack of deference' to the
Establishment. He reminded us that Mr Blair's supporters are fond
of saying that he listens as well as leads, but this time it was the
Maddocks who were doing the leading. 'Neither came across as a
political obsessive or a compulsive complainant. This was not the
pushiness of privilege, but something more straightforward and
compelling. The Maddocks family were simply no longer prepared
to tolerate the second-best which has been the hallmark of British
public services for decades.'

He went on, 'They genuinely could not see why, as tax-payers,
law-abiding citizens and loving parents, they should have to put up
with inadequate treatment for their daughter.'

D'Ancona had also spotted what many journalists find in the
couple: their skill in giving interesting, entertaining, yet informed
and above all inspiring television contributions. 'In their television
interviews, they were the soul of politeness. But there is not a shred
of deference in them. Not a scintilla... The couple is awesomely well
informed and well briefed. Twenty years ago, a family in their

predicament would have put jam jars on the counter of their local pub, inviting punters to donate their loose change. But the Maddocks couple run a website, have made themselves medically literate and – above all – are completely underwhelmed by politicians.'

Rival politicians were to recall the Blair encounter, too – for their own ends, naturally. The Conservative's shadow health minister, Dr Liam Fox later described that edition of *Question Time* as 'Tony Blair's humiliation'.

* * *

While admiration for them was transformed into newsprint in the small hours, the couple only managed four hours' sleep in their hotel. They were soon back in action feeding the broadcasters' ferocious appetite. Their first interview was for Radio Four's *Today* programme on the phone from their room. Then, without time for breakfast, they found themselves, shattered and a little fuddled, in a taxi bound for GMTV's studios on the South Bank.

Dean reflected that they were now 'riding a mad bandwagon'. He had no complaints. 'We set it off. We're on it now. We have to keep riding it to the end, to get the publicity to find the donors to help Alice.'

But would their remaining energy last out? By now the couple felt like chewing their clothes. They hadn't been within sight of food since *Question Time*. Even then, neither had been able to eat because of their butterflies. This breakfast television company had learned, aptly enough, how to make delicious first meals of the day. They laid on a mouth-watering array of orange juice, bacon rolls, croissants, marmalade, tea and coffee. And for a few rare minutes, Dean and Carol attacked the goodies before them. They were still eating when some other GMTV guests came over for a chat. Members of the Pop Idol group Hear'say seemed really interested in Alice, and promised to give her bone marrow appeal a plug whenever they could. 'We found them very nice, really sympathetic,' Carol recalls. 'But of course Alice would be thrilled that we talked to them, even if they'd tried to murder us.'

Carol also felt warmly towards Eamonn Holmes, GMTV's star presenter, who talked to them about the previous evening's encounter with Mr Blair for a good ten minutes – a long time on breakfast television. 'We were sure that after that interview, thousands more people would be encouraged to join the bone marrow register,' she said. 'Eamonn certainly did his best to pester everybody to sign up.'

But they didn't stay at GMTV long enough to find out if there'd been a hearty response or not. They were too busy hurtling out of the door and into a car sent by the rival BBC Breakfast News. After they'd done the interview at the TV Centre in Wood Lane, they followed up with more radio programmes – including one for BBC Radio 5. And still the mobile phones cried out for attention. As the media frenzy continued to fizz and buzz, the studio appearances, radio interviews on the phone and chats with newspapers and magazines dissolved in a seamless whirl in their harassed minds. They can't recollect exactly how many interviews they did. Or for whom.

To save creative energy, I'd told them to give the same answers to everyone. All seasoned interviewees do this, not just on the same day but for year after year. Journalists expect it and nobody seems to mind writing or recording the same old stuff. But the couple always forgot what they'd just told the last interviewer. And they were forced to think up answers anew.

People who have never been interviewed think it's as easy as pie. You just tell it as it is, don't you? Well, no, if you've any sense, you don't. Dean and Carol had learned you edit what you say as you go along. And in this present vortex of media interest, they wrestled hard to put their compact experience into practice.

* * *

They were aware, for instance, that reporters are trained (though they rarely admit it) to tease out as much sensation as possible. Sensation is everything. The ordinary mum who has a stand-up fight with Tony Blair in front of millions – and wins. The angry young husband unswerving in his support. Alice's state of health – is she getting worse? Here they are, folks – this is what the family looks like. That's about it. In the eyes of a hack journalist, the 'Alice Story' is not much more than entertainment. There are exceptions, of course. More 'serious' reporters bolster the sensation with 'educational' background material, even if the average person stops reading after the third paragraph.

Dean and Carol strive to put a different message across to the journalists. The just want to say that Alice needs a bone marrow transplant and please be good enough to sign the register. But they also knew that the *Question Time* incident was the big election story of the moment and without it there would be no more Alice coverage for some time. Dean said, 'Tired though we were, we knew we had to say the right things, to keep it simple, and above all to weave in a big appeal for donors.'

He didn't find this easy. 'During each interview, my stomach was in knots. Though we tried to smile to the cameras, we were struggling inside to find things to say to help our cause. We were skating on thin ice. Just one wrong word could give the wrong impression and switch people off.'

More than anything else, they strove not to let anything slip that would upset Alice, as she watched or listened with her grandparents back home. The reporters athe story of a mum and dad challenging the Prime Minister to save their daughter from an early death. But even if the subject of death needed to be raised on *Question Time*, it had to be avoided afterwards for Alice's sake. No easy task during an interview, where it's easy to let your mouth run away with you, especially when you're near exhaustion.

'We just wanted to go home,' Dean admitted. 'But we knew we couldn't. We had to stay until the last reporter asked the last question. As soon as this latest story was cold, they would drop us like a hot spud. We'd come across this burning need for topicality before. We just had to make the most of the Blair incident, because to be honest, I didn't think he would ever think about us again.'

With a start, Carol realised they couldn't stay in London for much longer. She remembered that Alice was booked in for yet another blood transfusion in hospital at teatime that same day. They did their final TV interview around lunchtime, refused a few later ones and shot off back up the M1. There was no respite in the car. Carol did more interviews on the move with national newspapers, the *Yorkshire Post*, *Yorkshire Evening Post*, *Dewsbury Reporter*, and scores of local radio stations. While still a hundred miles from Hanging Heaton, they realised they were never going to reach home in time to take Alice to hospital. So they arranged on the mobile for Alice's grandmother to take her and, just before the transfusion, Dean and Carol were reunited with their daughter at St James's Hospital.

The couple returned to worrying news. Alice's blood count was found to be much lower than expected. Once again, she was rushed back to hospital with a rocketing temperature. Over the next few weeks, she needed many more transfusions to stabilise her condition. Yet despite this extra burden and the continuing demands of the media, the couple went straight back into their local campaigning activities. The lights stayed on in their home as they toiled into the small hours, writing letters and emailing anyone who might be able to help. For the next few months, if they had one night a week off, they were lucky.

A Wrong Impression

Carol and Dean are far too sensible to run themselves into the ground. The time had come for a break, a chance to take their noses away from a huge grindstone and review progress so far. They fancied an old-fashioned seaside holiday, especially to please the girls. But they couldn't go too far in case Alice needed more urgent blood transfusions. So they packed for a week's holiday on the Yorkshire coast, staying in Dean's parents' new caravan. It was a happy choice. They thoroughly enjoyed their few days under a rare north-eastern sun. Alice's illness was forgotten as, despite the inevitable presence of a few reporters, they all made sandcastles, sucked seaside rock, paddled in an icy sea, sat around on deck chairs and behaved exactly like any other family would. But this happy break had a bizarre aftermath that made Carol boil with fury.

A month or two after the family's week away, a friend gave her a cutting from the *Sunday Express*. It was an advertisement for a competition to win a family holiday in Florida. The piece was dominated by a photograph of Alice, looking healthy and happy, lolling on a beach in what was obviously meant to be an exotic location. There was no mention of her illness.

On closer inspection, it was clear that the picture was actually of Hornsea, a pleasant but unsophisticated seaside resort near Bridlington in East Yorkshire. Carol recognised the picture as one taken by an *Express* photographer who had covered their recent holiday.

'I was affronted,' said Carol. 'They were giving two bogus impressions, neither of which was very nice. People would think I was using my desperately ill daughter as a child model. Even worse, the promotion made it look as though she'd made a full recovery, and that would stop donors from coming forward.'

Still smouldering, she rang me for advice. Meanwhile, Sally Wheeler from Express Newspapers marketing department telephoned to apologise to Carol. Shortly afterwards, she wrote to say the picture editor had gone to all lengths to make sure Alice's photo was not used again for advertising purposes. 'We apologise for any distress caused. I sincerely hope that Alice makes a full recovery.' I later spoke to Sally and found her to be a kindly woman who was very unhappy at what had happened. By now, I regretted trying to stir up press interest.

The *Express* was as good as its word. They did take steps to stop the photo being used again, and removed details of the holiday promotion from their website. They printed this apology in both papers:

'A competition in the *Daily* and *Sunday Express* to win a mobile phone and family holiday featured a picture of a smiling young girl. The picture was of Alice Maddocks, who has been bravely fighting a campaign to find a bone marrow donor and whose face is now widely known. The picture came from our library and its use was not intended to cause any difficulty or embarrassment to Alice or her family. We apologise to them if any has been caused.'

The *Express* also added to this message a footnote that really pleased the Maddocks. It was a plug for their website, inviting anyone with an interest in Alice's progress to log on.

Encouraged by the *Express*'s willingness to put things right with a full apology, I attempted to milk a little bit more from the incident. I asked their solicitor for modest compensation – 'say, about £2,000' – for the Alice Rose Trust. He asked about it, but we were turned down.

The Letter That Made Carol Jump for Joy

Dean had doubts about the Prime Minister's promise to meet them personally to discuss Alice's illness. He never thought for a second the pledge would be honoured. Surely, he argued to his wife, if Mr Blair were sincere, he would have approached them as soon as *Question Time* came off the air. He would have had a brief chat, confirming his intentions. Instead he'd walked quietly away. But Dean's doubts were very shortlived. The very day after the broadcast, a letter was sent to the couple from the Labour Party headquarters at Millbank in London. It was from Labour's Chief of Staff, Jonathan Powell.

'The Prime Minister was very concerned about your daughter's illness. It must be a very worrying time for you... I know that you have ideas on how the National Blood Service can improve its service and increase the number of donors...' But it was the next few words that made Carol scream with delight. Sitting on the bottom step in her tiny hall, she read, 'The Prime Minister would like to have a private meeting with you to discuss this...'

Carol couldn't continue. She felt sick with excitement. To challenge the head of the British government to do something about your problem on a prime time television special was the chance of a thousand lifetimes. But to get a letter saying the Prime Minister wanted to meet you to discuss your ideas face to face seemed like a miracle. Their ideas! To be considered by the Prime Minister! How about that!

But typically for Carol, she began to look for snags. Was this perhaps an election gimmick? Just an opportunity for Mr Blair to appear to be a thoroughly good bloke? A sneaky chance to win a few more votes? The rest of the letter put that suspicion to rest.

'To avoid any suggestion that the Prime Minister is seeking to exploit the case of your daughter for electoral purposes . . . he thinks it best if the meeting takes place after the election. Our office will be in touch with you after 7 June (Election Day).' Carol couldn't wait to have words with Dean, especially 'I told you so!'

Though it was Mr Blair's genuine wish not to exploit the story, somebody connected with him seems to have confirmed to the BBC the meeting would happen. On the day the letter was written, but hadn't yet arrived at the couple's house, the Prime Minister's intention to meet the Maddocks was reported on the BBC's website.

Back in Hospital

With the *Question Time* incident behind them, you might expect fate to give some respite to the Maddocks family. But there was no let up. In fact, nothing that had gone so far prepared them for the difficulties facing them now. Their new trials began when, with Alice's blood count showing no signs of improvement, 'Dr Mike' decided that yet more treatment was required to suppress her immune system to stop it attacking the bone marrow.

The couple had an uneasy feeling about this second round of hospital treatment. This was multiplied a few days before the medication was due to start, when Alice developed a patchy red rash around her stomach area. Her parents phoned the doctors and they all found themselves in St James's Hospital a day early. Alice had a case of shingles. It's caused by a virus that needs a healthy immune system to see it off. The trouble was that Alice's natural protection had been weakened by the previous therapy. So the new medication had to be put off until shingles had been treated and vanquished.

Dean and Carol were almost relieved. They knew from last time that the drugs to be used against Alice's immune system would cause fever, vomiting, headaches, diarrhoea, bruising and rashes. But at the same time, they wished fervently that Alice hadn't got shingles either. The condition could be fatal in Alice's weakened state.

The couple came home with Alice in a state of despondency; convinced that nothing pleasant would ever happen to them again. But when they checked their answerphone they found a message from the manager of S Club 7. Alice was invited to meet the band personally whenever it was convenient.

The news seemed to help. The shingles brought no complications and eventually subsided. So Alice returned to St James's for her anti-immune therapy. This time, the main drug, anti thanacite globulin, had been developed inside rabbits. During Alice's last long stay in hospital, the principal medication came from horses. Although this latest treatment would be very similar, it was hoped a slightly different drug might, just might, be more beneficial.

* * *

At least they thought so. But then came disturbing news. Doctors came to the difficult decision that Alice's liver was not strong enough to cope with the new drugs, after all. It was likely that Alice's recent attack of shingles was the culprit; it had stopped the liver working properly. The medics were very sorry but the treatment must now be put off again, and the family should go home. Meanwhile tests on Alice's liver would be carried out and the main treatment could start as soon as the organ was strong enough.

The Maddocks didn't have a chance this time to consider whether the reprieve was a blessing or not. Because as they prepared to leave St James's, the pains in Alice's joints got worse. Her temperature began racing up. She was plainly not fit to return to her cosy bedroom back home. Instead, she and her parents had to stay in hospital overnight. Dean and Carol didn't sleep. In their worried minds was the depressing thought that if just one hour's test dose made Alice so ill, what would the full course do to her over four weeks?

The couple now did a strange thing. They prayed that a woman they'd never met wouldn't have her baby when she expected to. She was the wife of 'Dr Mike', Alice's consultant. Their initial worries that he seemed too young for his job had long since vanished, replaced by a very deep respect for his skill, care and wisdom. His wife was expecting a child in the next two weeks. But Dean and Carol were praying the birth wouldn't happen till Alice had finished her treatment. 'We knew it was selfish,' said Carol, 'but we half expected the drugs to go horribly wrong and wanted "Dr Mike" to be on hand if they did.'

Dean and Carol floundered in a morass of acute anxiety. They felt far more apprehensive about this second round of treatment than when doctors had first tried it a year ago. It was easy to see why. Alice had been seriously ill after the last treatment to subdue her immune system. Added to that, some exploratory tests on the new drug she was to receive had already made her unwell. And this time round, the frailty of her liver was an added problem. They did their best to brace themselves for the horrors ahead, but the world seemed a hostile place.

* * *

If they could only find a donor, these aggressive anti-immune treatments would no longer be necessary. So during the waiting the couple continued their publicity crusade. Earlier, Carol had cancelled an interview for *That's Esther* because of the imminent hospital treatment. But when it was delayed, she contacted the production team to say they could take part after all. Technicians hastily arranged a link from the Maddocks' home to Esther's studio in London.

After the programme, a stream of concerned friends and relatives rang up. They all asked Carol how she was. They said things like, 'Oh dear, Carol, what's happening to you? You're doing too much. You want to pack it in while you still have your health.' Carol was puzzled because she didn't feel that drained. But apparently, everyone had been shocked at her appearance on television. She'd looked anguished, her face screwed up in what appeared to be terrible misery and she was slurring her words. Alice's illness was seemingly taking a greater toll than anyone realised.

But Carol was able to put her friends at ease. It wasn't the exertions of the latest episode in hospital that had made her look like a nervous wreck on *That's Esther*. It was the fact that the TV link between her home and London had developed a technical hitch during the broadcast. The result of this fault was that everything Carol said came back through her earphones in a series of disconcerting echoes. They prevented her from hearing what she was saying next. She was involuntarily screwing up her face to hear what the interviewer's questions were. And she was slurring her sentences because the sound of her own voice reverberated in her skull. In short, she looked and acted deranged.

'I wasn't at all pleased,' said Carol, who'd tried to look her best throughout the family troubles, mainly to reassure Alice, but also to demonstrate to the world that she can cope. 'I felt a right idiot. I don't know what people must have thought about me.'

Her sister Sue told her. 'They'll think you're on tranquillisers, that you've hit rock bottom and that you're at the end of your tether.'

'Thanks,' said Carol.

But eventually, though not for some time, Carol had to laugh.

* * *

Then, ten days after she was sent home from hospital, the doctors pronounced their satisfaction with Alice's liver and she went into hospital to start her delayed treatment. The schedule was daunting. First the little girl had a series of blood tests and transfusions. The drugs were injected at teatime. Three hours later Alice was feeling very unwell ... and 'Dr Mike''s wife went into labour.

Carol said: 'I was very, very frightened by that news. Who would fit into "Dr Mike"'s shoes? We had built up this terrific rapport with him. We trusted him. And I just resented his wife so much. I felt he belonged to us, not her.'

Dean was the same. 'How dare she, how dare she do this on the first day of Alice's treatment?' Both were mollified however, and a little ashamed of themselves, too, when another very capable consultant, Dr Sally Kinsey, took charge. She would be on 24-hour call in case Alice suddenly became worse.

Strong support was also on hand from another quarter. As soon as they were allowed, the loyal army of friends and relatives began visiting – and never stopped. As soon as someone turned up whom Alice knew very well, Carol and Dean would slip away for a cup of tea or a stroll in the hospital grounds. They couldn't stay away too long though as Alice could react traumatically to the drugs at any second.

That first session lasted from 6 p.m. until 3 p.m. the next day. During this long and harrowing period of 21 hours, Alice couldn't sleep. Her head throbbed, she kept being sick and was repeatedly carried off to the toilet with terrible diarrhoea. While this was happening, 'Dr Mike''s wife gave birth to a baby boy, whom they called Matthew. The news was brought to Dean and Carol who forgot all about their unworthy wish about the doctor's baby. 'We couldn't be more pleased when we heard,' said a penitent Carol.

The next morning, even though he'd only just started paternity leave 'Dr Mike' surprised everyone by popping up at Alice's bedside. Though lying in a torpor Alice raised herself weakly when she saw him. Dean and Carol noticed how tired the young doctor looked and were grateful he'd taken the time to come. It reminded them just how dedicated the staff on St James's children's ward were. And it was at this grateful moment that ambitious seeds were set in Carol's mind. She vowed then and there she would, one day, do something to improve the impoverished surroundings he and his loyal assistants had to work in. That undertaking – huge in scale and ambition – was to start in less than a year's time, but for now the Maddocks' priority was to see Alice through the immediate crisis.

The Boy Who Didn't Come Back

Of course, Alice wasn't the only patient on the ward enduring torment and anguish due to some more aggressive forms of medication. Many brave toddlers, children and teenagers were fighting the harsh side effects of chemotherapy for various cancers. It was more than enough for Dean and Carol to bear their own daughter's distress, without watching other young people lying prone and in pain, surrounded by drips and other intimidating pieces of hospital paraphernalia. Carol and Dean knew they had to concentrate all their efforts on Alice if they were to bring her through, so they forced themselves to ignore the pitiable scenes around them. They weren't always successful.

In the middle of the night, Carol was dozing when there was a sudden commotion around the next bed. A ten-year-old boy's heart had stopped. Curtains were quickly drawn around him, but the sounds of his parents' distress and the intense activity of doctors could be heard clearly. Carol, terrified for the little boy, could only hold her breath. She overheard that he needed to be moved to intensive care. But that area was about ten minutes' walk away, down a few levels and along many corridors. His attendants decided it would be dangerous to make the transfer. So for two hours, Carol listened in tense trepidation as attempts were made to resuscitate the child. This was awful! Carol wondered how she could help, then realised there was nothing to do but pray for the little boy. Eventually, the doctors managed to stabilise his condition enough to move him on a trolley to 'intensive care'.

In the morning the little boy's parents returned to Ward 10. They looked underneath his bed and emptied his bedside locker. They didn't seem to want to talk, and Carol daren't ask about their son. She watched them sorrowfully. They went away without looking back. To Carol it seemed like a heavy silence had descended. The usual hospital sounds, children's voices, vacuuming, clattering crockery, were no longer there. Alice's voice, squeaky with her illness, broke the silence. 'Where's that boy gone?' Carol told her that he was very ill and had been taken to a different part of the hospital where nurses could look after him a bit better.

All that day, Carol wondered what had happened. In the evening, she asked 'Jolly Trolley', the auxiliary nurse, if she'd heard anything. For some strange reason, she found herself whispering. 'What's happened to the little boy who was in that bed?'

'Jolly Trolley' breathed back one word, 'Died.'

Carol was shocked. Soon afterwards she resented the staff for not telling her this sad news earlier in the day. 'I was mad with them for not respecting me enough to come and tell me. I know all about the duty of confidentiality, but I don't think it would have hurt to let me know, just the same.'

Later on, Carol reasoned that the staff must constantly face many sad incidents. It was part of their normal working life. They were not keeping secrets. They just hadn't thought it was important for other parents like Carol to know.

But they should have told her nonetheless, because Carol and Dean had long ago come to terms with the possibility that 'it might be their turn next'. Said Carol, 'If I had been told, with ordinary sensitivity, what had become of that poor little boy, I could have accepted it. Telling us would have helped us to cope with horrible events that might be ahead for our family as well. Instead we learned of it in a whisper, as though it was some big, awful secret.' She added, 'All I could think of when I found out, was how can we get Alice off the ward before it happens to her?'

* * *

It was because of tragic incidents like this, happening all around them, that the couple tried to get a side ward as they'd done before. But this time there wasn't one available. In fact, the main ward seemed less equipped than during their previous stay. Even essential things were now in short supply. Though the couple had a folding bed to snatch some rest during Alice's gruelling treatment, they couldn't find blankets or a pillow for it.

Dean is meticulous, partly by nature and partly because of his training as a policeman, and he'd brought last year's diary with him

to the hospital. In that diary was a daily record of the drugs Alice
had previously taken and the times they'd been given. He'd also
noted down those drugs that had been more effective than others.

'This put us more in control than last time,' said Carol. 'We were
able to go up to the nurses and say it's time Alice had this drug or
time she had that done, and so on.'

Dean didn't think the staff were too happy about this. 'I suspect
they had us down as interfering busy bodies. But it wasn't true. We
just wanted to give Alice the best chance possible, by making sure
the treatment went exactly as it was supposed to.' Carol however
thinks differently, 'I believe the nurses were secretly happy we were
putting our oar in, because they were so busy.'

During the long hospital days, Dean again made himself busy in the
kitchen, trying to cheer up his wife with culinary magic on the two-ring
cooker in the ward's tiny kitchen. Every evening, round Alice's bed,
they tucked into one of his special salads and a glass of wine.

'This time, we had the uncomfortable feeling that some of the
other parents thought we felt we were a cut above them,' Carol said.
'But we weren't. We were just trying to bring a bit of our normal life
into the hospital.'

Half way through the treatment Chloe, in the care of Dean's parents,
was taken ill. She had trouble breathing. The doctor put it down to mild
asthma, and she was given a nebulizer. Everyone believed that stress
was the cause. Chloe was fretting over Alice and missing her parents.
Meanwhile, Alice was getting worse; her bouts of sickness were
became more frequent and the pain in her joints increased. Thankfully,
a side ward was now free and she was moved into it.

* * *

At that time, there were lots of promotions for the National Lottery
on television. The jackpot, swollen by a week's rollover, stood at
£17 million. Alice had been given morphine for her pain and,
affected by the drug, couldn't stop rambling about the big prize. 'If
I won all that money I'd build a special laboratory,' she told her
mother, 'to make everybody here better.'

She elaborated on the theme. 'This lab will make everybody in our
family, who has died, come alive again. And we'll all live together in

one big house. And the garden will have sweets in the flowerbeds. And there will be a fairground in the garden, free to all poorly children.'

Alice talked about her plans for the lottery money all morning. But then she became very ill with painful diarrhoea. Throughout the night, every half-hour or so, she was taken to the toilet. She was also sweating heavily and her shoulders were extremely painful; the serum sickness was coming even earlier this time. This was uncommon and proved how sensitive Alice's body was becoming to the toxic drugs.

Dean and Carol were now very worried. Was the cure worse than the disease? However, this time round they felt much more able to cope with the situation and knew the side effects would pass. But their many questions were temporarily forgotten when senior consultant Sally Kinley came to Alice's bedside and started everybody laughing with her opening words, 'Hello, have you got your grandfather visiting you, Alice?' The 'grandfather' was in fact, Carol's comparatively young brother-in-law, Richard. Even Alice chortled. Day by day the side effects subsided and Alice was eventually allowed home.

The family came back to a message on the answering machine. It was from Downing Street. Would they make an appointment to see the Prime Minister on 23 July? This was exciting news – but just the same, the couple were apprehensive. They knew, from their earlier experience, that treatment to subdue the immune system could bring delayed side effects. If those kicked in, this vital meeting with Tony Blair would need to be cancelled. It was one more thing to worry about.

No Tea, Thank You

Carol nursed a big worry about the vital meeting with Mr Blair: 'What am I going to wear?' She considered she couldn't work out any strategy for dealing with the Prime Minister until this little problem was put to rest. With close friend Sarah Walsh, acting as consultant she drove to Sheffield for an intensive shopping trip. Within ten minutes of searching, she chose a snappy suit in cornflower blue, with navy shoes. The next seven hours were spent in an exasperating hunt through dozens of shops for a dark blue top to go under the suit. The two women, footsore and frazzled, never found one. Carol arrived home in a temper, only to discover in her wardrobe a forgotten inky blue top she'd never worn. Sarah, of course, was not told the embarrassing truth.

Dean and Carol were determined not to miss a trick in their meeting with Mr Blair. Every angle had to be covered, every eventuality foreseen and planned for. Nothing must go wrong, for Alice's sake. But they were seasoned campaigners now and the task didn't daunt them. So as not to appear as lone voices, they decided to hand him a petition stiff with the names of ordinary people supporting their crusade. Both spent a day, with the blessing of the management, in Sainsbury's in Dewsbury. They put up their faithful electronic notice board and displayed leaflets and posters in the entrance hall. Brandishing clipboards and looking businesslike, they took hundreds of signatures from shoppers, most of whom already knew Alice's story and wished them luck. At the same time, local newspapers carried petition forms for their readers to sign. These were sent by hand to the Maddocks' home. Another large bundle of names was also delivered – of nearly every policeman and woman in Bradford.

Dean and Carol had studied all the literature available on their subject and felt ready to answer anything Mr Blair might ask. But to be on the safe side, they asked one other person to go with them to Downing Street. The British Bone Marrow Donor Appeal is a charity that raises cash for the National Blood Service, helping it to maintain the Bone Marrow Register. The Maddocks asked this charity's leader, John Humphries, to join them. They were impressed by his knowledge of the bone marrow issue, but mainly they wanted the Prime Minister to hear from the horse's mouth how the National Blood Service had to go cap in hand to a charity for money.

We expected Downing Street's press office to alert the media. But Carol and Dean didn't want to rely on that. Two weeks before the event, I rang round to forewarn health correspondents on the newspapers, radio stations and TV stations. There was plenty of interest. Many producers began ordering clips of *Question Time* for yet another chance to show that celebrated moment when Carol savaged Mr Blair.

Nobody was surprised that some journalists couldn't wait for the meeting and went into print early. The *Sunday Mirror* dressed Alice in a white doctor's coat and photographed her holding a first aid box. With this smiling picture was the headline: 'WE DON'T NEED ANY TEA, MR BLAIR, JUST HELP US TO SAVE OUR BRAVE ALICE'.

This was a reference to Carol's powerful quote in an article by journalist Sheron Boyle detailing how she would not be letting the Prime Minister off the hook.

'We don't want tea and biscuits at number 10. We know that his [the Prime Minister's] time is precious, and even more so for Alice. The drugs Alice takes can cause her serious damage, so the quicker a bone marrow match is found, the better.'

* * *

The BBC's breakfast television show rang up to ask the couple to appear on the morning of the big day. I counselled against it. This meeting was too important to waste nervous energy on a speculative interview that might irritate Mr Blair. Rather than spending time with journalists, the Maddocks buckled down to some intense preparation. They wrote a three-point agenda for the meeting. Each section came with a full page of explanation – how Alice was diagnosed, the hunt for a donor and how they wanted the Prime Minister to help. They worked long and hard into the night on this document. They regarded it as the turning point in the fight for Alice's life. Journalists who've seen the Maddocks' document afterwards have marvelled at its clarity, accuracy and style. It puts to shame those judges and academics who write high-powered reports for the distinguished departments of Whitehall.

But while serious preparations for the meeting went on, media fixers asked for yet more interviews. Researchers on the BBC and GMTV breakfast shows pressed for all they were worth, offering hotels, chauffeured cars and long appearances in prime spots.

Anyone experiencing this kind of thing knows how seductive the inducements can be. But Dean put his foot down. 'I had to be really firm with them. We were not getting up at some awful hour just to help them out. We were convinced this meeting with Mr Blair would save Alice and stop her suffering for good.'

It may be easy for some to label the Maddocks as self-seeking publicists, but it wouldn't be true. They never have and never will let the media spotlight outshine their dedication to Alice's wellbeing. They always make their daughter's health their first priority. Proof of this came a few days before their meeting in Downing Street. Results of tests just received showed that Alice had a very low platelet count. So Dean took her to hospital for two more blood transfusions. By the afternoon, Alice's face was swollen and she looked very unwell. Both Dean and Carol prepared, sadly but determinedly, to call off the meeting with Tony Blair. But Alice, as she so often does, fought back. Not because she wanted to save the meeting in Downing Street, but because she had a big role in a school play.

Looking a bit better, but not much, Alice went back to school the next day. Carol was also there, painting the faces of Alice and all the young performers in her class. And on the eve of the big London trip Mum was again back on school duty – this time making fairy cakes for the end-of-term party. 'I don't know how we're getting through all this,' she wrote in her diary.

Dean in Danger

Though Carol was working too hard, Dean was undergoing an even tougher strain. In fact, not long before their visit to Downing Street to see the Prime Minister, he found himself fighting for his own life. One hot Saturday, word came through to him from Bradford police station that all officers were needed at once. They'd been told that rioters were getting ready to attack the city. Dean obeyed the call. He was ordered to tour the streets in a people-carrier with two other officers. They were looking for outbreaks of trouble to report back to headquarters. All seemed fairly quiet, despite an ominous gathering of hundreds of people in front of the Town Hall. Suddenly trouble broke out. There was fighting between anti-Nazi supporters and members of the National Front. A young man in the angry crowd was critically stabbed. Then the fury was transferred to the police.

Dean and many of his colleagues found themselves at the wrong end of flying stones, iron bars, bottles and half bricks, not always fending them off successfully with dented riot shields. As a policeman went down, he was carried to safety by running medical teams. Flying objects were injuring scores of officers. Eleven hours now after he first came on duty, Dean was exhausted, yet the riot was becoming even more violent. A large crowd came together in the White Abbey area to the north of the city. Frenzied youths were hurling petrol bombs and setting cars alight, pushing them towards the police. 'We were getting hammered and injured with everything they could throw at us,' recalled Dean.

Under a fog of acrid black smoke, the police formed into a long row, which the rioters tried to force backward with a rain of missiles and burning cars. These flaming vehicles, their hand brakes off, were shoved down sloping streets towards the thin blue line. Officers were forced to shuffle backwards in retreat. As they lost ground to the advancing horde, rioters were able to recover missiles they had hurled earlier, and throw them again. Trying to protect a police cameraman, Dean was hit on the head with a brick. Only his reinforced riot helmet saved him from brain damage.

'Another policeman would fall beside me every two minutes. I had some amazing escapes, expecting at any moment to be burned to death by flying petrol. I was terrified.'

Working among the police was a press photographer whom Dean recognised. Only the day before, he'd been having tea and sandwiches, after taking pictures of Alice in the Maddocks' garden. 'We just looked at each other and shook our heads in disbelief. A few hours was all that separated a sunny tea party on the lawn and a murderous riot,' said Dean sadly. 'It seemed to reflect our life with Alice – one day exhilarated by brilliant news, the next hurled down by something unspeakably bad. It's a barmy world!'

Gradually though, the police got the upper hand and the attackers trickled away. Four hundred officers were seriously injured that night. Dean was relatively unscathed with only an injured toe. He arrived home at 4 a.m. after more than 24 hours at full stretch, defending the peace from screaming rioters. For many months now, he'd struggled to stay on police duty, while caring for Alice and campaigning for donors. But the riots were the final straw, proving to him that he couldn't do all three jobs at the same time. He felt he must let his police superiors know he couldn't carry on for the time being. Although he feared their reaction, he had no need to. His boss told him to take as much time off as he needed. Relief flooded his mind. He was now free to tackle Mr Blair on full power.

Downing Street

The pair had arranged to stay in a London hotel so they could set off on the afternoon before the glorious 24th, have a long night's sleep and be as fresh as a mountain stream for the big meeting. They would need every second of that sleep because the preceding day was extremely strenuous. Dean went into work at Bradford police station in the morning, while the unsinkable Carol did interviews with Yorkshire Television, BBCTV, the two nearest local radio stations and three newspapers. In view of all their support so far, she felt she couldn't refuse. But after the manic activity of the last few days, by early afternoon, the couple still hadn't packed. Everything they needed for an interview with the most important person in the land, was part of an untidy pile on their bed, with Dean's blue three-piece suit, the only decent one in his wardrobe, lying crumpled on the floor. Dean's mother Joan was coming round to collect the girls. The minute she arrived, she was pounced upon and asked to pack the bags.

As the car pulled into the road three hours later than planned, Carol was in a state of frenzy. 'I'd no idea what Joan had packed for us. Had we got everything? Had she remembered my lipstick, my nightie, my posh shoes, the new blue suit? I like to be organised to the last detail, and we certainly weren't. We were losing control.'

On their way down I rang the couple. 'Don't let John Humphries hog the show.' True, John had many years' experience of hard work with the British Bone Marrow Donor Appeal, but he'd never had a meeting as important as this. I've never met John, but I've encountered many old-stagers in the charity world and they tend to be talkative. I reminded Carol and Dean that this was their show, the result of their extraordinary effort. The eyes of Britain were on the woman who had bested the Prime Minister, not anybody else. To make the most of this rare opportunity, the Maddocks must not be upstaged. Dean and Carol told me they'd already considered my fears and told me not to worry. They'd a lot of time for John Humphries and assured me he would be very useful in dealing with Mr Blair. As it turned out, they were absolutely right.

* * *

Later that evening in a swish London hotel, where they were staying as guests of GMTV, the Battling Maddocks were being whispered about. Staff and guests cast furtive looks their way. Carol was evidently recognised as the woman who'd badgered Tony Blair during the election campaign. But the gossip was tinged with respect, not hostility, and the couple found they were treated like VIPs. Fellow guests smiled and said 'Good evening' more than usual. Waiters and receptionists were excessively courteous. Bags were spirited away to their rooms and no one hovered for tips. They were provided, free of charge, with an expensive reception room for any television interviews they might want to do. Taking my advice not to tax themselves in London, they'd agreed to do only one interview that evening – with GMTV.

They had dinner at the hotel with Matthew Taylor, a *Yorkshire Evening Post* reporter who'd covered Alice's story from the beginning. Now relaxed, for perhaps the first time in a week, they began to realise the enormous importance of tomorrow's meeting at Number 10. There was also time for pessimism, and Dean gave way to it. 'Everybody knows what politicians are like and I thought we were expecting too much. I was beginning to feel we hadn't an icicle in hell's chance of getting anything out of Mr Blair. I thought the best we could hope for was for him to say, "Thanks very much and I might get back to you – eventually."'

Finally alone, the couple trudged to their room. But wearied though they were, they couldn't relax. Dean recognised his wife was on the brink of collapse. He knew that, though friends regarded Carol as a tower of strength, she had a breaking point. And he feared this was just around the corner. He even entertained the fear she might have some sort of breakdown before dawn came. 'Oh no,' he thought selfishly, 'I'm going to have to see the Prime Minister on my own.' Carol caught the same cynical mood.

Once between the sheets however, she began to resume her usual confidence. Even so, the couple didn't talk to each other. Both needed silence after such a frantic day. They mulled over their desires, anxieties and fears about tomorrow's meeting. Dean still brooded bleakly to himself in the dark, 'I just know Mr Blair is going to dismiss our views as nothing to do with him. And if he does show us the door, where the hell do we go from here?' He turned over and over on the bed. 'We've been through the local blood service, through their national office, to government ministers, the local press and the national papers. If he turns us down tomorrow, we've nowhere else to go.'

Dean was now very low. They'd gone further than all other bone marrow campaigners in the past. If they fell at this last jump, then he was ready to give it all up. After all, they had two wonderful daughters to care for, one desperately ill, and both needing their love. Both Dean and Carol needed more time to provide it.

Still awake, two hours later, Dean found more strength of purpose. Though it was unlikely that Mr Blair would meet all their wishes tomorrow, surely he would at least promise to think them over. And if Mr Blair did that, Dean reflected, they could be satisfied, and perhaps return to a more normal life, away from flashing cameras and prying TV lenses. That would be a lot better than this current life of struggle and disappointment. Finally he slept.

* * *

It was a short night for the Maddocks. Two hundred and twenty miles away in Tenby, I imagined reporters gathering round their hotel like wolves. Though I'd asked the couple to fend off the media, rather than exhaust themselves before the big meeting, I made an exception for Radio 4's *Today* programme. In fact, two weeks earlier I rang their planning desk to suggest they talked to Carol and Dean early on the day of the Blair conference. My reason was that I expected Mr Blair to be listening to the BBC's flagship programme. More importantly, the opposition would be tuned in. If the Prime Minister didn't come up with the goods at the 'big meeting', then I was ready to stir up a media outcry. Doubtless, the Tories and Liberal Democrats would be delighted to join in.

The Maddocks talked to the *Today* programme. They had a good slot, beginning the first half of the programme, just after the seven o'clock news. They skilfully handled a longish interview with no critical questions. The presenter seemed fully behind them. That done, the couple went down to breakfast. A bit later, ITN turned up at the hotel, together with a crew from the *That's Esther* show.

The news crew were acting a bit strangely. They appeared to be interviewing somebody else in the hotel foyer. Curious, Carol asked what they were doing. 'Talking to the Anthony Nolan Trust,' said the soundman. Afterwards, Carol introduced herself to the new interviewee. She thought she seemed a bit sheepish. To tell the truth, the Maddocks were a bit put out that ITN had brought this woman from the Anthony Nolan Trust to their hotel. As usual when somebody snatches a publicity victory, there are others in the same field happy to share the limelight, not for egotistical reasons, but to snatch some of the publicity spoils for their own organisation.

I'd previously warned Dean and Carol about this understandable tendency. It was the same temptation I feared might presently be facing John Humphries. By now the couple were becoming worried that others might try to muscle in on their critical get-together with Tony Blair. Who else had been invited to Downing Street that they didn't know about? Would they be prepared for what these other visitors might say? The appearance of somebody from the Anthony Nolan Trust at the hotel reinforced their concern. Carol wasn't even sure the charity was fighting for the same things. 'We'd had a lot of contact with the Anthony Nolan Trust, had joint donor sessions with them, and they didn't seem to want any involvement by the government at all,' she explained. 'They preferred to stay independent, as they had done for 25 years. For the Trust's representative to talk about our meeting with the Prime Minister seemed very odd to us.' But they shrugged off the incident and set off for Downing Street on foot.

They didn't take a taxi because someone at the hotel said Downing Street was 'just around the corner'. Much to Carol's dismay because her new shoes pinched, it turned out to be quite a long walk in blistering July sunshine. During it, television crews continually filmed the couple from the front, the sides and behind. Being part of such a conspicuous procession was unnerving. They felt they had to appear confident of success for the sake of the turning cameras. This called for a constant smile and a rather jaunty way of walking. But by now, Dean's shoes were hurting as much as Carol's and the city's heat was overpowering. Because of the constraints of filming, they couldn't even walk in the shade. They were very relieved when they strode painfully into Downing Street.

There were scores of reporters and cameramen at the heavy black gates barring the public from the street. This eager throng was swollen by just as many tourists who assumed that Mr Blair was expected shortly, or at least a member of the Cabinet. In the confusion, Carol and Dean were swamped by questions from reporters. They fended them off rather brusquely, because by now they were worried about the time. 'Never be late for the Prime Minister,' Carol told herself.

Dean fumbled in vain for the Downing Street letter to prove who they were. Giving it up, he approached the bobby on the gate. The smiling policeman said, 'Certainly... this way,' and swung back the gate into Downing Street. Then came a 100-yard walk to Number 10. More policemen and women were standing along the way. Each one knew why the Maddocks were there, and wished them luck. 'I was very stirred by that,' said Carol. Opposite the best-known terrace house in the world, Dean glanced to the left where he saw an even bigger herd of reporters, photographers and interviewers. Dean was exhilarated by the sheer size of the media cohort. But it was only a few seconds before the buoyant mood evaporated and his heart sank again. The same old worry was back, 'What happens if he refuses to help? What are we going to tell this lot? Do we get angry or do we accept it with good grace?' He remembered that I'd told him to make an almighty fuss if Mr Blair let them down. But could they do that to the Prime Minister? He had, after all, been kind enough to see them. This nicety wasn't a worry for Carol, though. If Mr Blair let Alice down, he would receive from her the colourful public lambasting he would richly deserve.

* * *

There was just time for the couple to answer a few more questions from the reporters, some holding notebooks, others poking mini recorders at them. 'It was all very jolly, very friendly,' according to Dean. News photographers asked them to pose in front of the famous door and then knock on it. Dean beat on the door in a theatrical manner for the cameras. He was just about to do it again for luck when the door swung open and the couple found themselves standing on the large chequered black-and-white flags of a splendid hall.

They were shown into a reception room, which to their surprise was full of people. It was a grand room, with a large desk at one wall. They were asked to leave their phones and camera on it. From here they were led to a smaller waiting room. This retreat had a marble fireplace, elegant dining chairs and paintings around the walls. It also had ordinary net curtains through which they could peer out into Downing Street.

'Can you imagine the strange feeling for us?' asked Dean. 'We were at the most prestigious house in Britain, not just looking at it, but actually inside and looking out,' he marvelled. 'We couldn't get over it.'

They could see the restive crowd of media people lurking about outside. Carol had a pressing impulse to pull aside the nets and wave to them all. The temptation was so strong she actually stood up to do it. But Dean, keen to preserve the dignity of the occasion, urged her to stop fidgeting and sit down. He had no trouble sitting quietly himself. Running through his mind was the thought of all the famous people who'd graced this same antique chair over three centuries. Foreign ambassadors, heads of state, kings and queens – and now Dean Maddocks of Dewsbury. But he reminded himself that few of those past occasions could have compared in urgency to the battle to save Alice.

The five-minute wait seemed like a couple of hours. Dean's palms were damp, his mouth dry and his stomach jumpy as he struggled to control the attack of stagefright that had begun when he woke up that morning.

A woman's head popped round the door. After introducing herself as Katie Kay, one of Mr Blair's aides, she said, 'The Prime Minister is ready for you now.' 'Just like going to the dentist,' Carol thought. As Katie escorted them down an endless corridor, she congratulated the couple on their achievements so far. She'd seen their bravura performance on *Question Time* and 'admired' them for it. 'Mr Blair is a very nice man, so there's nothing to worry about. He will listen to you.' Two hearts lifted as one.

As they walked, they passed impressive paintings and sculptures, each one probably worth more than their house in Hanging Heaton. But Carol wasn't interested in her sumptuous surroundings. She could see Alice's drawn but smiling face in every portrait, on each marble bust. Her mind sneaked back to St James's Hospital where her daughter had an appointment that same day. Just about now, she would be setting off from home with Dean's mother. Even though this was a routine visit to hospital, Carol still felt guilty about not being there – neither parent had ever missed one of Alice's appointments before. She had plenty of time to worry about her little girl. The walk, in her tight, squeaky new shoes, went on and on. They processed up and down different staircases, along more corridors and through picture galleries. It was clear that 10 Downing Street was much more spacious than it looked from the outside.

At last, they were shown through double doors into a vast room with windows overlooking the garden. About a dozen people were working at desks. From there, they were shown into a connecting smaller room. It was furnished with striped Regency sofas and chairs, a couple of three-legged wine tables and a carved marble fireplace. This was a room where touring visitors were never allowed – Tony Blair's office.

John Humphries, dark-suited and distinguished, was already in the room and there was somebody else that they knew. It was Dr Angela Robinson, of the National Blood Service, the woman Dean had accused on the *Today* programme of not doing enough to find bone marrow donors to save Alice's life. She gave them a smile that was not at all wintry. In fact, despite their past differences, the couple were rather glad that she was present. Dean had found she 'gave a straight answer to a straight question'. There were others in the National Blood Service whom he felt did not deal so competently with them. Dr Robinson was never patronising. But nevertheless he feared that today she would still take the old line that everything was fine with the bone marrow register, and nothing else needed to be done. If she did that, and Mr Blair believed her, then they were sunk.

There were perhaps a dozen more people present, secretaries to take notes and grey-suited officials from the Department of Health and the Treasury. Tony Blair was already sitting down, but he rose and walked across the room to greet them.

Carol shook his hand and began, 'I'm very sorry, Prime Minister, for shouting at you.'

'No, you mustn't be sorry,' he smiled. 'I would have done exactly the same thing.'

Carol was struck by the way Mr Blair looked directly and steadily into her eyes. She'd found this quality very rare among doctors, health officials, politicians and journalists. She immediately trusted him. 'He's going to help us, after all,' she thought brightly.

'I was going to offer you some tea,' said Mr Blair, 'but I read in the papers you're not here for tea and sympathy. [Journalists had told the Maddocks that the trouble with Mr Blair was that he talked a lot, offered tea and sent people away with vague promises. This is why Carol had given her 'no tea' quote to the *Sunday Mirror*.] Anyway, I hope you'll change your mind and have some tea, because I'm absolutely parched.'

Carol said, 'We only told the papers that about the tea because we wanted you to know we're here for very serious business,' adding, 'but yes, we'd love some tea.'

The couple found themselves on one settee by the fancy fireplace, facing the Prime Minister on another. He first asked, 'How's Alice?' then added, 'I understand she has a sister. How is she coping with all this?' They were impressed. Everybody inquired about Alice, but to be concerned about Chloe, who'd coped so well with the mound of attention lavished on her sister, revealed, they thought, a considerate nature.

Dean was pleased when Mr Blair insisted that the couple should open their discussion together. They were used to people from the National Blood Service snatching the first word. Carol told him about Alice, their fruitless hunt for a donor, what they thought was lack of commitment by the health authorities and the need for money for a larger bone marrow register. She told him that parents and charities should not have to bear the lion's burden of finding more donors, but that the National Blood Service should be much more active in the search. The need for more donors from ethnic minority groups was even greater. Tony Blair listened carefully. Then he turned to health officials and asked if the National Blood Service wasn't already trying to recruit as many donors as possible.

Dean expected a spirited defence, a haughty denial, but they weren't offered. Instead he was astonished at the honesty of the replies. The health officials, standing in the background, meekly agreed with the Maddocks that they didn't have the resources to do justice to sick children like Alice. Tony Blair seemed unhappy at this. And after each new accusation by the Maddocks, he became more and more perturbed. He kept turning to Angela Robinson for an explanation. And she continued to agree that the couple were telling the truth. 'It was a rhapsody to my ears,' said Carol.

Then came some more music from Mr Blair, 'So what do we need to do to bring this service forward?'

Dr Robinson from the National Blood Service began, 'Well, we're doing all we can...'

Carol, ahead of the game as always, exclaimed to herself, 'Good grief, he's asking you what you need. And you're not telling him. What you need, is more money!'

But unfortunately, Dr Robinson wasn't telling Mr Blair that. She was proudly informing him that 17,000 new names had been found for the bone marrow register that year. Dean was indignant. Most of those people had come forward after campaigns by amateurs like themselves, including Molly-Ann Barnett's family, and many other parents and well-wishers. The National Blood Service could claim very little credit for finding any volunteers at all. As far as Dean knew, the service had run no publicity campaigns or advertisements whatsoever.

Mr Blair was plainly on the Maddocks' side now. He wasn't at all satisfied with the answers he was getting. At one stage he declared, 'This isn't good enough!' Carol was amused to hear him echoing her own words from *Question Time*. She clearly remembered telling him, 'It's not good enough, Mr Blair!'

It was now obvious the Prime Minister didn't want to hear what the blood service had been doing until now; he wanted to know how things could be bettered. He asked again what was needed here and now. Again Dr Robinson began to repeat her last comment.

This time Carol couldn't help herself. She cried aloud, 'For goodness sake! What you need is more money!'

And Dr Robinson replied that it was true; they couldn't move forward without extra resources.

'In that case,' promised Mr Blair firmly, 'it will be provided.'

Silence. This was remarkable. Dean thought, 'These are my lucky numbers coming up on the lottery. It can't be true, can it? This is everything.'

Carol quickly turned to her husband. Her face was creased in delight, the dark patches under her eyes gone. 'We just wanted to cheer. This was our highest goal and we had won it. It was wonderful, wonderful!'

For a moment John Humphries looked as though he was about to cry. But instead he asked, 'Does this mean top slicing, Prime Minister?'

'Certainly,' replied Mr Blair. Onlookers nodded sagely.

But Dean had a quietly worded question about this, 'What's top slicing?' It was explained that 'top slicing' meant a grant of money to be paid directly by central government. The money would come with no strings attached, no going cap-in-hand to local councillors.

The couple thanked Mr Blair profusely. Carol couldn't help apologising again for haranguing him on television. 'But we had to do it,' she told him, 'for the love of Alice and for the love of all those young people in this country and around the world who need bone marrow. We couldn't bear to think of one more family going through what we've been through.'

'Sometimes,' Mr Blair laughed, 'ordinary people have to make a fuss. Sometimes that's how change comes about.'

Dr Robinson was as pleased as everybody else was. She told the Prime Minister that the National Blood Service would now set a target of 40,000 new donors a year. Dean wondered if he should take a leaf out of Carol's book and haggle for more donors – say 50,000 names – but immediately changed his mind. They'd already gained so much. A target of 40,000 was, after all, eight times the number of volunteers added to the register only two years ago. Carol also decided not to press for more jam on the bread. For once, she was content.

Cheerfulness and joviality entered the crowded room, replacing formal courtesy. There was universal satisfaction at the outcome. The business side of the meeting was over in 40 minutes. But an amiable Prime Minister chatted to the Maddocks for longer. He asked about Alice and Chloe again. Carol inquired about his baby son Leo. Dean suspected Mr Blair was wondering how he might feel if Alice's fate befell a member of his family.

The subject of 'teenage years' cropped up. 'Don't talk to me about the teenage years,' laughed Mr Blair, though he didn't elaborate. 'It was just like gossiping to another parent at the school gates,' Carol recalled.' We tried not to be overawed by Mr

Blair. After all, our business with him was the most important imaginable. But when the horse-trading was over, it seemed quite wonderful that the busiest, most powerful person in the land was nattering to us about everyday problems with kids.'

It was Carol who wrapped things up. Pleasant though this once-in-a-lifetime encounter was, she couldn't wait to bring the news of victory to the waiting press pack. Pulling Dean along, she almost ran through the great rooms and corridors towards the grand hall. They launched themselves through the front door 'like kids on the last day of term', according to Dean. 'We were beaming. We'd got far more from Mr Blair than we'd ever dreamed possible.'

Reporters struggling to catch their first words mobbed the pair. Television news teams didn't finish with them for nearly three hours. Dean in particular was keen to do every interview on offer, because at the back of his mind, a nasty little warning was taking shape. They had nothing in writing from Mr Blair. Cynically, and at the same time ashamed of the thought, he reasoned that by sending their good news into millions of homes, the Prime Minister could never change his mind.

The couple accepted an invitation to go on BBC Breakfast News next day but only if the corporation could organise accommodation – they were learning fast how these people worked. When they jumped into a cab to the Kensington Hilton, a favourite with the BBC, the driver said, 'I've just seen you two on the telly.' He acknowledged their fighting spirit and would not take anything for the £20 cab fare. 'I admire you for what you've done,' was all he said.

They called the girls to tell them that they'd had a wonderful time and that the Prime Minister was very nice and would help Alice all he could. They learned in return that Alice's blood count was now especially low and that she was very ill.

Alice is Very Ill

Good news and bad are soul mates in the tense saga of Alice Maddocks. A lesser family would simply not be able to withstand the stresses caused by constant, sudden displacement of good luck by ill fortune – and vice versa. They are always going to hell and back in very short spaces of time. Although Mr Blair's promise to increase the funding for the bone marrow register had buoyed them up, Carol and Dean were now deflated by dark tidings about Alice's health.

A sombre-faced 'Dr Mike' gently told them that he'd reviewed the case with a professor at Great Ormond Street Children's Hospital in London. Both experts were worried. They would not reach perfection with Alice. She was not in remission and was never likely to be. Alice must continue with the drugs to suppress her immune system. Long-term use of these can lead to further serious medical complications such as organ failure, further damage to her immune system and cancer. However, to take her off these drugs would mean her being dependent on blood transfusions; this they could not risk as it would lessen the chances of a successful bone marrow transplant should a donor be found.

They had also considered a third course of treatment to try and suppress the immune system. Like the previous two rounds of treatment at St James's, this regime would stop immune agents in Alice's blood attacking her bone marrow. However, both experts feared that a third round of immunosuppressants would put too much strain on Alice's weakened constitution and might be fatal. In any case, the first two attempts hadn't made much difference.

'Dr Mike' went on to say that no new donors had been found, but they would continue to search. Just like Alice's parents, they would never give up hope.

Once more they were thrown back on their desperate hope of finding a donor with the same tissue type as Alice – not just similar, not even very similar, but identical. Yet all the searches so far, made all over the world, still hadn't found one registered donor able to help. This made their campaign to encourage more people to sign up more vital than ever. But how long could the couple fight? The strain, now more than two years old, was nearing breaking point.

After hearing the latest verdict that no drugs would help, Carol confessed to *Yorkshire Post* news reporter Alex Buller, 'People look at us and think we are really strong. But living with all this uncertainty all the time is destructive. We get on with our lives, and Alice goes to school, but it never leaves our minds that aplastic anaemia, bad though it is, might soon turn into something else. If that happens, doctors will tell us that Alice has only got a few weeks to live.'

From Mexico with Love

Into the cramped hall in the Maddocks' home dropped its most distinguished letter yet. Tony Blair had written personally to say how glad he'd been to meet them. 'I was very sorry to hear about Alice's illness and the problems she faces.' He praised their clear explanation to him of how the bone marrow service could be improved. 'As well as wanting to help Alice, you also want to help other children in a similar position. I found our discussion on ways of improving the bone marrow registries very useful. And I am pleased to tell you that the National Blood Service has now agreed to accept bone marrow samples from new blood donors throughout the country.'

He confirmed that he'd agreed to all the couple's demands for improvements. The most important change would be a £6 million present to the National Blood Service 'to enlarge and service the bone marrow registry'. This extra cash would treble the size of the bone marrow register. The Prime Minister ended his letter: 'Please give my best wishes to Alice. I do hope she continues to remain well despite the rigours of her present treatment.'

So now it was official. The cautious Dean had the 'Blair Promise' in writing. It wasn't until he had self-indulgently read the letter three or four times that Dean noticed something odd about it. It was widely travelled. From a few words printed at the top, it was clear the letter had first been written by Mr Blair while he was on holiday with his family in the resort of Cancoon in Mexico. From there it was faxed to Downing Street and then forwarded on to the Maddocks' home. So, Dean realised, the Prime Minister had interrupted his cherished summer break just to keep the Maddocks informed of progress. 'We were really flattered,' said Carol. 'It was evidence of how anxious he was to rush things through – just for Alice. We knew from our meeting that he was keen to help, but this proved to us how really committed he is. That letter meant so much.'

* * *

Seven weeks later, Mr Blair's senior policy adviser, Simon Stevens, sent a four-page report to the Maddocks. It was one the Prime Minister had asked the Department of Health to prepare on ideas to expand the bone marrow registers. The note that came with it was friendly and helpful – a mile away from the rather cold tone of the letters Dean and Carol had from civil servants before *Question Time*.

Simon Stevens concluded, 'This report picks up key points from your meeting with the Prime Minister, and work is now taking place in conjunction with the relevant organisations. We will of course keep you fully updated, but please let me know if I can be of any help in the meantime. Best wishes.'

Though the Maddocks had sparred with the National Blood Service over the last two years, its directors hold no grudges. In fact they're delighted at the outcome of the couple's campaign. 'We are extremely grateful,' they told me. 'We now have the money to put 40,000 new donors on the register, and that wouldn't have happened without their meeting with the Prime Minister.'

Death of a Crusader

It was only a few weeks after the Prime Minister sealed his historic promise, that another famous mother in the unhappy world of bone marrow disorders sent a poignant letter of congratulation to Dean and Carol.

Thirty years earlier, Shirley Nolan's son had been born with a rare deficiency in his immune system. He had died at the age of seven after a fruitless search for a donor to save his life. While he was ill, his mother had set up, in his name, the Anthony Nolan Bone Marrow Trust. It was a pioneering organisation that went on to establish the first international register of bone marrow donors. And since then, Shirley Nolan OBE had never stopped trying to prevent other children from succumbing to her son's tragic fate.

Though she was now very ill, losing a long struggle against Parkinson's Disease, Shirley dictated a long letter to the Maddocks to thank them for securing Tony Blair's promise to revitalise the register she had begun all those years ago. Speaking was hard for her, but she dictated the message from her home in Australia to her sister Linda, who also happens to live in Yorkshire.

Shirley Nolan said she could 'now die with dignity', because her life's aim had been achieved – and that was thanks to the Maddocks family. Because of their efforts the Government had finally got the point of building up the register. The Maddocks found these words very moving. So much so that Carol even considered flying to Australia to meet her idol. But sadly Shirley died soon afterwards. Her legacy? Thousands of lives saved.

Alice's Tea Party

Mr Blair's tremendous boost to the bone marrow register made such a strong impression on Carol that it swam up and down her stream of consciousness for a long time. And as the anniversary of the Downing Street meeting approached, she wrote to Mr Blair with a progress report on Alice, and to thank him once again. To bulk out

this hymn to the Prime Minister, she added the fanciful suggestion
that he might one day like to meet Alice. But though she dismissed
the invitation as wishful thinking even as she wrote it, the reply, sent
in less than a week, was a thrilling surprise. Yes, Mr Blair would
love to meet Alice. Could her parents ring Downing Street to fix a
date? Carol and Dean were bowled over, gladly telling all their
friends and relations. But when a more formal invitation came in the
post, they discovered that the family was requested not to take tea
with Mr Blair at all, but with his wife Cherie.

All the euphoria of the earlier invitation evaporated. Carol was
seriously offended. She rang me in a sour mood, asking what she
should do. I suggested she rang Downing Street for an explanation.
There followed some stiff exchanges with the staff. Carol told a
secretary firmly that she wanted Mr Blair to see Alice for himself,
as he had done so much to help her – not his wife. Cherie, she
argued, hadn't been part of the story in any way. Downing Street
responded politely, but offered no alternatives.

Carol was later ashamed of making such a fuss. After all, the
Prime Minister was deeply occupied by affairs of state. Who could
expect him to spend vital business hours having cups of tea with an
ordinary family from Dewsbury? The girls could still savour the rare
opportunity of walking through that celebrated black door. And
Cherie Blair is worth meeting anyway. She is Britain's First Lady.

The Maddocks generously suggested that Molly-Ann Barnett
and her parents should be invited to the big tea party. Much to Paul
and Mandy's delight this was agreed by Number 10. So the two
families arranged to travel together by train and stay in the same
London hotel. The Barnetts were to bring the gin and the
Maddocks the tonic! As it was, Dean forgot the tonic and was
rewarded with a ticking off from Carol. He didn't care; he was
determined to enjoy himself.

On the couple's previous trips to the capital they'd been ravaged
by apprehension, hating the thought of crossing swords with health
chiefs, the producers of *Question Time* and the Prime Minister. It
had been hard physically and even more taxing of their minds.
They'd known that a wrong move could stop or start a chain

reaction that might cost their daughter her life. But this time, thankfully, there was no crude lobbying to be done – just the chance to relish a pleasant social occasion in fabulous surroundings. A tea party to remember!

They didn't think the news pack would bother them this time round. Even so, ten days before the tea party, I rang round all the usual editors, together with a few from the USA, Canada and Australia. Dean and Carol thought this was a waste of effort. Though anxious as ever to attract publicity in the relentless quest for donors, they couldn't imagine the kind of world-weary reporter they'd met would be interested in something as mild as a cup of tea at Number 10! I tried to persuade them otherwise. Their story was still hot. Mr Blair had grappled with the couple on television; now Cherie Blair wanted to have a jolly time with them. Parties and politics make a heady mix.

Though not convinced, Carol put on her thinking cap, searching for an angle to please the press. Choreographing the media was second nature now. She didn't have to rack her brain for long. She decided to re-run the old 'worry people' trick. These were the pipe-cleaner figures Alice had given to Prince Charles when he opened the Robert Ogden Centre at St James's Hospital nearly two years ago now. Tony Blair probably had more anxieties than anyone else did in the country, even the heir to the throne. So why not let Alice give a new set of 'worry people' to him? But it was Alice, innocent of the publicity value of her tiny creations, who developed the idea. With great secrecy, she set to work in her bedroom. This time, she made her pipe-cleaner models into replicas of the Blair family. She fashioned tiny bendy figures of the Prime Minister and all his children. The Cherie replica was holding the baby. With her pocket money, she also bought a wooden trinket box to put them in.

The 'worry people' would certainly be needed. The media engine rapidly fired up again. On the day before the Downing Street tea party, breakfast television fixers (a breed of TV people who attempt to set up interviews at all costs), news broadcasters, press reporters, the whole noisy lot of them, clamoured for more interviews and photos. At home, on an inter-city train rattling south and in their London hotel, the Maddocks' mobile phones jumped with calls. This time reporters knew that, for the first time, Alice was coming to London, and that made things even more interesting. Alice the resilient was not overwhelmed by all the attention and, while Dean and Chloe stayed in the background, she and her mother made the most of the interest lavished on them. They were rushed around radio and television studios in taxis and limousines and thoroughly enjoyed it. 'Everybody was so kind and considerate towards us', remembers Carol, 'that this time I really did feel like a queen for the day.'

* * *

Tired after a long morning and early afternoon of intense media activity, the two families each took a taxi to Downing Street. They hoped the ride would give them at least ten minutes of relaxed privacy. But inside the Maddocks' cab all was not well. Nearly there, Dean was aghast to find he'd left their signed invitation on the hotel bed. Meanwhile, their cab was going nowhere. There was a tube strike underway and that, combined with ambitious road works, had trapped them in the middle of a giant traffic jam. Time was getting short, making a return to the hotel for the invitation pretty risky.

Carol testily pointed out that she didn't think they'd be allowed into a security-ringed Downing Street without some kind of authority. So the driver was asked to head back to the hotel. He U-turned with difficulty and after a laboured crawl, the invitation was retrieved, and they stopped and started their way back towards Whitehall. During the tense journey, Dean studied the meter. He was perturbed to find it showed £40. Once again, and to Dean's secret relief, the driver, who already knew all about Alice, would not accept the fare. London cabbies may have big mouths, thought Carol, but they have hearts to match.

A gaggle of reporters surged on the foursome in Downing Street. But they were already late and couldn't afford any time to talk. Thankfully, they were spared that as, beneath its white fanlight, the famous dark door opened a fraction and they were hauled inside by an attractive fair-haired woman of about 35 called Fiona Miller. She was wearing a striking lilac shift dress with a long matching coat. Carol was taken aback by this vision of upmarket haute couture, and couldn't stop herself from saying so. 'What a beautiful costume. It really suits you.' Naturally enough, Fiona was flattered into talkativeness. As they all moved further into Number 10, their immaculate guide told the family how much she liked the way they'd challenged her boss on *Question Time*. Then she said something that made Dean and Carol even more pleased. 'Tony will be here this afternoon – especially to see you.'

This was an exciting surprise. Until this moment, the couple had expected to see only Cherie, even though they'd slyly hinted to the media that Tony would be present, too. Bubbling with anticipation, they were shown into a large room. A handful of other guests, in Sunday best, were already there. Between them, incongruously, moved a young barefoot woman in tracksuit bottoms. Following her around, was a little boy also shoeless and wearing a luminous turquoise T-shirt and blue shorts. It was Leo Blair with his nanny.

Dominating this stunning room, with its high vaulted ceiling, was a long antique table, capable of seating at least 60 people. Dean recognised this, from replicas in James Bond films, as the State Dining Room where the world's powerful and distinguished people were entertained. The Queen and Duke of Edinburgh had dined here on the eve of Winston Churchill announcing his retirement in 1955.

Fiona introduced Cherie Blair to the couple. Yet again Carol rushed to clear the air. 'I'm very sorry I shouted at your husband,' she began quietly. 'It's not something I take pride in.'

Cherie smiled. 'Don't worry,' she reassured Carol. And then, mirroring her husband's earlier words, 'It's only the people with the courage to shout who get heard.' It was at this moment that Carol's conscience finally stopped bothering her about the way she'd deliberately set out to embarrass the Premier. She never apologised to anyone about it again.

'Anyway,' Cherie asked quickly, 'how is Alice?'

Carol started. Obviously, Cherie didn't think the healthy-looking, smiling girl at her side could be suffering from any serious medical condition. She said, 'This is Alice.'

'Wow!' exclaimed the other woman. 'This is Alice? Why, Alice, you are beautiful!' Then she shouted to the toddler in the turquoise shirt, 'Leo, Leo, come over here. You must meet Alice!'

The Blairs' youngest son padded across and regarded Alice with huge eyes. He stroked her biscuit-coloured linen party dress and said 'pretty girl'. Chloe stepped up then and handed him a gift – a bag with a teddy bear inside. He grasped the bear and wiped its warm fur over his face. Then he secured the toy under his arm, backed away beaming – and ran off.

It was such an intimate moment between two families that Dean felt a strong desire to hare outside and shoo the reporters away. His musings were cut short when Tony Blair and a couple of security men entered the room.

Carol recalls, 'Mr Blair was also surprised when he saw Alice. He must have expected to see a worried, sickly, fragile child. But Alice often looks well, and this afternoon she seemed fitter than ever.'

The Prime Minister dropped to his knees to talk to Alice at eye level. 'He certainly understands children,' Carol thought. 'A family man.'

Return of the Worry People

Alice whispered to the Prime Minister: 'Hold out your hands. I've got something for you.' She placed the pipe-cleaner figures carefully in his palms. 'This is your family. You put them in this box. They don't make your worries disappear. But they do look after them for you.' Dean will never forget the startled look on the Prime Minister's face. 'It seemed he had been given an amazing insight into the meaning of life,' he said. 'A Downing Street photographer caught the moment and you can still see that emotional, quite shocked look in Mr Blair's face in the picture. It was fascinating.'

But Alice had already lost interest in the Prime Minister. Like little girls everywhere, she had an overwhelming desire to see what the toilets were like. Carol was curious, too; Fiona told them they were the same 'Ladies' used by the Queen on her many visits here. 'We left the Prime Minister and spent quite a long time in these loos instead,' Carol admitted. 'In fact, we didn't want to leave them at all.'

Apart from their meeting with the residents, the couple were deeply impressed by the Georgian splendour of Number 10, by the politeness of the staff and by the many different ways they were made to feel special. 'The whole visit was like our wedding day,' said Carol. 'We didn't want it to end. We tried to capture every second of our visit, so we could remember this fantastic, historic house in all its lovely detail.' Another thought struck her. 'You couldn't have a greater difference between this and our small semi-detached in Dewsbury, and yet Tony Blair and his wife were treating us as equals. That's what was so nice about them.'

As the family wandered about Number 10 in awe, Carol was somehow parted from the other three. She found herself ambling up the splendid main staircase on her own, overlooked by portraits of stern-looking former prime ministers. As she glanced up, she saw Tony Blair, flanked by bodyguards, walking towards her on the landing above. Heavens! What should she do now? Her father, a stickler for everyday protocol, would have advised her to 'bid him good day and go about your business'. This she decided to do. It wouldn't do to waste any more of this world leader's time. It belonged to the country, after all. As the two approached each other, it seemed to Carol like a film sequence in slow motion. She saw that Mr Blair was watching her. Then he stopped and asked, 'Can I have a word with you?'

'Perhaps I shouldn't be up here on my own,' she thought in alarm. 'He's going to tell me off.'

Yet the Prime Minister was smiling. 'Can you thank Alice for her worry people, Carol? It's the best present I've ever had.' The grin broadened. 'I've been handed some wonderful gifts in my time, but I've never been given anything like that. Tell Alice I'll put them on my desk and keep them there all the time. Tell her I will treasure them forever.'

The Prime Minister paused and looked thoughtful. Carol waited respectfully. 'But the only thing, Carol,' he added, 'is that I could have done with them ten years ago!'

He put his hand on the eighteenth-century mahogany banister, and leaned casually against the ornate metal supports. Carol relaxed, too. 'I found myself chatting away with him about family life, being a parent and life in general. He said how lovely it was that she'd given him the worry people. He remarked about how delightful young children are. I commented that we had the hardest times to come with teenage years and he jokingly replied, "Don't mention it. We're going through just that with our older son, Euan. Boy, has he given us some sleepless nights! It's difficult to know how to get it right because you never seem to be able to with teenagers."'

'We were two parents chatting about the children we love. He is good man, politics aside, a family man and that comes over quite clearly when you speak to him. I went on to thank him for his help in our fight to save Alice. I will never forget his response.

'"Sometimes, Carol, ordinary people make extraordinary changes. And quite clearly that is what you and Dean have done. You don't have to thank me." I was so moved by his remarkable comments.'

Mr Blair seemed reluctant to end the conversation. Later, Carol found it hard to believe what had happened. 'It was exactly like talking to Dean, or a brother or a good friend. Yet this was the Prime Minister. The last word for setting our taxes, changing our laws and starting and stopping wars!'

After what seemed like a very long time, they parted and the impassive security men again closed in around the Premier, leaving Carol to look for Dean and the girls. 'You've been gone ages,' said Dean mildly.

'Oh just having a chat with the Prime Minister,' she replied, studying his face for reaction.

'That's all right, then,' replied Dean abstractly. He'd just seen the room at which IRA bombers had fired a mortar shell during Margaret Thatcher's premiership and was apparently more interested in that.

* * *

Then the visit was over and they found themselves, with the Barnett family, back in Downing Street, doing more interviews. They couldn't concentrate on their answers though, because of a pressing physical need. They were all ravenous. They'd expected Number 10 caterers to lay on a full buffet of sandwiches, sausage rolls, buns and cakes. Instead they'd had a custard cream each and a cup of tea. 'Naturally we didn't eat before we went to Downing Street, so by the time we'd done our TV and press bit we were utterly starving,' Dean remembers.

Both families almost ran down Whitehall searching urgently for a café. They bought burgers and chips from a fast food place, and sitting on benches outside a pub, inelegantly wolfed them down. Carol found this very funny. 'One minute, tea and biscuits with the Prime Minister and his wife, the next burger and chips in a pub yard. Talk about a comedown!'

The big day wasn't over yet. Relying on their usual energy, the Maddocks had booked theatre tickets and they all piled into two cabs for the West End. With seconds to spare, they took their seats for *My Fair Lady*. Only Molly-Ann enjoyed the show. One by one, the rest of the party dozed off. Back at the hotel, the two Maddocks girls revived and began playing 'interviews' with Molly-Ann in the corridor outside their rooms. They took turns at pretending to be television reporters, their mums and dads and Cherie and Tony Blair. The parents were entranced by this noisy spectacle 'We just laughed ourselves silly watching them,' said Carol. 'It was a perfect end to our happiest day since the troubles began.'

For the Love of Alice

Leaves falling in central London. A youngish man, trim and smartly dressed, strides towards Waterloo station. He peers at his watch and quickens his pace. There's still no sign of his destination, though he knows it's around here somewhere, because they told him so at the hotel. He's not from London and hasn't yet learned that the locals never come to grips with the sheer scale of their city. When they give directions, saying such and such a place is 'just around the corner', they mean up to a mile away. Still no sign of the station. The walker breaks into a trot. It's getting late now and his wife is waiting for him at a big awards ceremony, now far behind him.

He's forgotten to bring a tie with him, you see. Somebody at the hotel told him there was a little shop open all hours in Waterloo station. At last he suddenly sees the station, and running very rapidly now tears into a tie kiosk. He grabs the nearest tie from a display and looms towards the counter. The only assistant is on the phone. Before she can end the call, Dean Maddocks throws down a ten-pound note, murmurs that he doesn't want the change or a receipt and hurls himself back into the jostling crowd outside.

Grateful for the fitness training for policemen, he speeds back toward the awards presentation like a greyhound after a rat.

The Maddocks had been invited to the prestigious Oyster Awards sponsored by the *Sun* newspaper, to honour campaigners who had helped to make changes to benefit the community during the year. At the glittering venue in a swish entertainment suite under the Globe Theatre, Carol also had a little problem to contend with. She'd just heard that Cherie Blair would be present – and she was wearing the same scarlet jacket she had on when she last met the Prime Minister's wife in Downing Street!

Half an hour before the 'and the winner is . . . ' moment, a refined voice behind Carol said, 'Do you mind if I sit down?' indicating a seat that Dean had just vacated to wander off somewhere. It was Cherie Blair.

'Please tell me how Alice is doing,' she said.

Carol explained that still no suitable donor had been found. 'She seems really shocked by that,' Carol thought. 'Cherie went on to say how she was in support of the use of cord blood for stem cell replacement and that she wished she had known about this when she had had Leo. She said it was an insurance policy and something all new parents should be aware of. I told her that Alice is now too old to receive cord blood and we had considered having another baby in the hope that a third child would be a perfect match for Alice.' Cherie was sympathetic. 'You are in such an awful dilemma,' she said.

Carol changed tack and told Cherie that she wasn't likely to win an award tonight, but if she did and had to make an acceptance speech, did she think Tony Blair would mind if she publicly thanked him for revitalising the bone marrow register?

Cherie beamed. Yes, her husband would be delighted... ' because he comes under such dreadful criticism – and something positive like that would make him so thrilled. So yes please, do thank him!'

'Well, it's so comforting to know now that everything is running much more efficiently, with much more chance of a donor for Alice. And without the Prime Minister's support... well, it wouldn't have happened.'

This pleased Cherie Blair. 'My husband really did feel for your case and he was greatly concerned about your daughter. Some people have a big impact on what the Prime Minister does and Alice is one of those people.'

The two women from such different walks of life chatted together until Cherie said, 'I must go. My pudding's arrived – and I do love my puddings!'

Carol didn't win the award. A doctor who counsels patients who've had difficult circumcisions and a man who campaigns for weekly payments to hospital patients took joint honours. This was rather to Carol's relief as she'd dreaded making a speech, especially to an audience that included luminaries like the Home Secretary, David Blunkett. After the ceremony Mr Blunkett's bodyguard came over to Dean to tell him, 'I can't believe your wife didn't win. You've both done so much for children.'

* * *

The ordinariness of the Family Maddocks that began this book has disappeared forever. Like Shirley Nolan before them, they will be a huge influence in the future on the health of Britain and indeed the rest of the world.

People in their home county of West Yorkshire have recognised the family's amazing achievements. In the summer of 2002, Carol was invited to the Yorkshire Woman of the Year lunch organised by the *Yorkshire Evening Post* (YEP) and held in Leeds. 'I thought I was invited as a guest of my good friends at YTV's news programme, *Calendar*. The speaker began talking about this unnamed woman whom I didn't recognise. I was trying to work out who she was but was impressed by her achievements. Then when my name was mentioned, I was rooted to my seat. I blushed furiously and couldn't believe when it was announced that I'd won the YEP's Woman of Achievement Readers Award. As I stepped up to the stage, I just wished Dean was there and thanked God that I'd bought something new for the do! I didn't feel deserving of it but was thrilled by it and it means a lot to us as a family.'

Meanwhile, Alice gained her own award when she won a Yorkshire Young Achievers Award and was presented with it in front of an audience packed with sports and TV stars. 'She was thrilled with it. The event was an excuse to buy a new dress, but she still understands that the award is for all that is being done for herself and others in her name,' says Dean.

And the Alice Rose Trust, started so reluctantly will, given the Maddocks' tenacity and energy, be a beacon in the lives of all families who have seriously ill children.

Though Alice's life still hangs on a thread, and their care for her never ceases, Dean and Carol have embarked on another massive project – to build a new children's hospital to serve the whole of Yorkshire. The campaign for such a centre is not new, but it has floundered for the last fifteen years. Needless to say, the Maddocks have given it new life. Their enthusiasm stems from all the anxious days they've spent in Ward 10 at St James's Hospital. It was then that they made promises they would fight for better conditions for doctors and nurses to work in. They also want to put an end to the present fragmented system where sick children and their families are shunted around the city for different treatments and tests.

'One big hospital for children, with all the comforts of home,' says Carol, 'that's what our children and all the doctors and nurses deserve!'

With all the Maddocks' experience of dealing with authorities and raising funds, the hospital will surely come into being. Senior hospital staff, MPs and parents of desperately ill children have already swung behind the battling Maddocks in their towering ambition.

* * *

All the considerable effort by Dean and Carol to find the right donor for Alice has failed. Yet paradoxically their work has been a stunning success. The National Blood Service's bone marrow list is now the fastest growing register in the world – with a target of 40,000 new donors a year. Presently the seventh biggest register, it's now on course to become number one in the next few years. And if it weren't for the Maddocks, many patients with leukaemia and similar blood diseases would have died. The couple have encouraged many thousands of people to go on the registers and have forced the Government to put much more money into the National Blood Service. They have revitalised, publicised and greatly swollen the register, not just for the sake of this country, but for the world. We owe them a great deal. Meanwhile the search for a donor for Alice goes on.

'Alice has good days. Her condition has stabilised due to the heavy medication she receives on a daily basis. Her spirits are higher than ever and we try to run as normal a family life as possible – for both our daughters' sakes,' says Dean. 'Since Alice became ill, we have gone through horrendous times but it has been a humble learning experience. But we pull together as a family and our fight continues for Alice,' says Carol.

Carol believes the past few years have given them many happy memories too. 'We have discovered things about ourselves which we didn't know. We're stronger emotionally than we realised. The girls are very compassionate and understanding of people's needs. They have been through a lot and have seen things that you would not choose for them to witness but they are growing into loving and thoughtful young people.

'I know the irony of the situation. I know we have saved many people's lives by our work. But the knowledge that we have not found a donor for the person we most want one for lives with us every minute of the day. Alice is our lovely, brown-eyed, intelligent daughter with a thirst for life. Her witty comments crack us up with laughter and her constant singing drives us crazy at times.

'We have two beautiful daughters and we look forward to seeing them both grow into beautiful women. And so, Dean and I will continue our fight to find a suitable donor – for the love of Alice.'

Easy steps to becoming a bone marrow donor

1) Ring the National Blood Service 08457 711 711.

2) Ask for the time and place of the next blood donor near your home.

3) Go to the session to give blood.

4) Before you give blood, ASK to register as a blood marrow donor. If you are already a blood donor, you should still ASK to register as a marrow volunteer.

5) An extra sample of blood will be taken to assess your marrow. Your name will be entered on an international register.

6) Wait for the call, which may or may not come.

Alternatively, ring the Anthony Nolan Trust on 020 7284 1234. They will send you an information pack on how to become a marrow donor. However, the National Blood Service route is the quickest and is of course an opportunity to give blood as well.